CANCER ETIOLOGY, DIAGNOSIS AND TREATMENTS

METASTATIC MELANOMA: SYMPTOMS, DIAGNOSES AND TREATMENTS

Cancer Etiology, Diagnosis and Treatments

Additional books in this series can be found on Nova's website under the Series tab.

Additional E-books in this series can be found on Nova's website under the E-book tab.

CANCER ETIOLOGY, DIAGNOSIS AND TREATMENTS

METASTATIC MELANOMA: SYMPTOMS, DIAGNOSES AND TREATMENTS

SARAH A. KLEIN
AND
JAMES P. BECKLER
EDITORS

Nova Science Publishers, Inc.
New York

For permission to use material from this book please contact us:
Telephone 631-231-7269; Fax 631-231-8175
Web Site: http://www.novapublishers.com

Library of Congress Cataloging-in-Publication Data

Metastatic melanoma : symptoms, diagnoses, and treatments / editors, Sarah A. Klein and James P. Beckler.
p. ; cm.
Includes bibliographical references and index.
ISBN 978-1-61209-915-6 (hardcover : alk. paper)
1. Metastasis. 2. Melanoma. I. Klein, Sarah A. II. Beckler, James P.
[DNLM: 1. Melanoma--secondary. QZ 202]
RC269.5.M485 2011
616.99'477--dc22

2011004606

Published by Nova Science Publishers, Inc. † New York

Contents

Preface

Melanomas are usually highly proliferative, invasive and are most frequently metastatic. Melanoma accounts for nearly 4% of skin cancer cases but, because of its highly metastatic capability, for 74% of all skin cancer mortalities. Therefore, melanoma is one of the deadliest forms of cancer and its treatment continues to be challenging. This new book presents topical research in the study of the symptoms, diagnoses and treatment of metastatic melanoma. Topics discussed include new therapeutic alternatives for melanoma; the metastatic cascade and experimental treatments; pediatric melanoma and the relative risk of metastatic melanoma.

Chapter I – The incidence and mortality rate of cutaneous melanoma have been increasing more rapidly than any other cancer over the last three decades. The leading cause of mortality in melanoma patients is metastasis formation. Thus, it is necessary to find treatments that can block metastasis to improve survival of melanoma patients. The production of metastases is a highly complex process by which some melanoma cells move away from the primary tumor and colonize other organs. This process requires phenotypical changes that allow melanoma cells to migrate, survive in the blood circulation, extravasate, and proliferate in a tissue with a different microenvironment. Accordingly, new therapies aimed to block metastasis must target cellular functions like adhesion, migration, invasion, and homing. Having a different mechanism of action than cytotoxic and cytostatic drugs, such therapies could be used in combination with the current ones. This chapter reviews some key signaling pathways that affect melanoma metastasis and discusses the targeting of those pathways in different preclinical models. Such strategies may become the basis for the generation of new therapeutic alternatives for melanoma.

Chapter II– Cancer is a major health problem and is the second leading cause of death in the world. Invasion and metastasis are the greatest obstacles to the successful tumour treatment. Metastasis is a multi-stage process involving adhesion of the cancer cells to the basement membrane, invasion through the basement membrane, cancer cell motility, intravasation, transit in the blood or lymph, extravasation and growth at a new site. Any drug, which can inhibit one of the steps in the cascade, will be useful in the inhibition of tumour metastasis. Death from cancer is most often due to metastases that are resistant to conventional therapies. Although there are several drugs available to encounter cancer growth in humans, there are no drugs presently available to specifically inhibit the metastasis of cancer cells. This review focuses on metastatic cascade and possible therapeutic targets.

Chapter III – Melanoma is a malignant tumour originating from melanocytes (cells responsible for generating melanin, the pigment that gives colour to skin, hair and eyes). This pigment is the strongest in moles. It is due to this reason that melanomas are usually brown or black in colour. Sometimes, melanomas stop producing the pigment and appear red, pink, and even skin-coloured.

Chapter IV – An international panel, comprising a cross section of expert melanoma surgeons who have contributed data and leadership to further investigate the role of sentinel node biopsy (SNB) in melanoma, recently produced a consensus statement, outlining their overall interpretation of current evidence, as a guide to clinical treatment of patients with clinically localized melanoma. They agreed that SNB is standard of care in current practice because it is incorporated in staging guidelines from the AJCC, incorporated in the treatment guidelines from the National Comprehensive Cancer Network, and practiced by most specialty surgeons who treat melanoma in the United States, Australia and Western Europe. The proven benefits for performing sentinel lymph node biopsy at the time of oncological wide local excision of a primary cutaneous melanoma in any patient, include both prognostic and staging information, the potential therapeutic impact of a completion lymph node dissection in those with a positive node and also has implications of nodal status for adjuvant therapy decisions or entry into pertinent clinical trials.

The prognosis for patients with a thick cutaneous melanoma (Breslow thickness >4 mm) is poor, with a 10-year melanoma specific mortality rate >50% and 5-year disease-free survival of <50%, causing both treatment difficulty and uncertainty for doctors, as well as patients. Because of this poor prognosis and high degree of synchronous metastatic disease at initial presentation in patients with a thick primary melanoma, the approach to the regional lymph nodes remains extremely controversial. The high risk of synchronous distant metastases is suggested by some to outweigh any benefit of staging or the possible therapeutic benefit of elective lymph node dissection in this group of patients. However, a significant amount of these patients survive without recurrent disease. Detection of lymph node involvement in thick melanomas may help to identify this group, particularly given that other factors (ulceration and Clark's level) seem to have less prognostic value in this group.

The aims of this book chapter are (1) to examine the possible prognostic and therapeutic role of sentinel lymph node biopsy as a potential standard of care for thick melanoma, (2) to evaluate the results of pertinent clinical trials and whether they can be extrapolated to thick melanomas and (3) to critically assess other emerging strategies targeting this difficult patient population.

Chapter V – Controversy concerning whether pregnancy portends a poor prognosis for women diagnosed with malignant melanoma (MM) has led to questions concerning the effect of exogenous hormones (hormone replacement therapy, oral contraceptive pills) on MM prognosis.

Since the 1970's, many epidemiologic studies have attempted to address the impact of oral contraceptive pill (OCP) use and relative risk of MM. Far fewer studies have addressed the influence of hormone replacement therapy (HRT) on relative risk of MM or on prognosis in those diagnosed with MM. Herein we review the history of the controversial relationship between hormones and MM, and analyze the relevant studies. Overall the evidence to date does not suggest a link between exogenous hormones and a woman's risk of developing MM.

Chapter VI – Cutaneous melanomas are the malignant and aggressive tumors of skin with extremely poor survival rates for the patients diagnosed with locally invasive and metastatic disease stages. Despite intensive research has led in last few years to an improvement of the curative treatment of early-stage cutaneous melanomas by tumor surgical resection, ionizing radiation, systemic chemotherapy, immunotherapy and/or adjuvant stem cell-based therapies, the locally advanced and disseminated melanomas are generally resistant to conventional therapies and result to the death of cancer patients. The rapid progression of primary melanomas to locally invasive and/or metastatic disease stages remains a major obstacle for an early effective diagnosis and a curative therapeutic intervention for melanoma patients. Importantly, recent advances in the melanoma research have led to the identification of different gene products that are frequently implicated in the malignant transformation of melanocytic cells into melanoma cells, including melanoma stem/progenitor cells, during cancer initiation and progression to locally advanced and metastatic disease stages. These oncogenic events include the occurrence of activating mutations in distinct oncogenes such as v-Raf murine sarcoma viral oncogene homolog B1 (B-RAF) or neuroblastoma RAS viral oncogene homolog (N-Ras). The enhanced expression and activities of diverse growth factor signaling elements such as epidermal growth factor receptor (EGFR), sonic hedgehog, Wnt/β-catenin, Notch and vascular endothelial growth factor (VEGF)/VEGF-R receptors in melanoma cells also represent common molecular events associated with melanoma progression, metastases at distant sites, treatment resistance and disease relapse. Of therapeutic relevance, these deregulated signaling transduction components constitute new potential biomarkers and therapeutic targets of great clinical interest for improving the efficacy of current diagnostic and prognostic methods and management of patients diagnosed with locally advanced, metastatic and/or relapsed melanomas.

Chapter VII – Purpose: Uveal melanomas typically metastasize to the liver. A sensitive and specific serological marker for metastatic disease would be of great value. The small globular protein "melanoma inhibitory activity" (MIA) is established as a marker for cutaneous melanoma. This study was performed to evaluate MIA as potential serological marker for early detection of metastatic disease in uveal melanoma.

Method: In a prospective study, we collected serum samples of 390 patients with uveal melanoma. Serum samples were analysed by using a one-step enzyme-linked immunosorbent assay (ELISA) to quantify the MIA serum levels. All patients also underwent standardized A-scan echography to measure the maximum tumor height.

Results: 31 (7.9 %) patients had proven metastatic disease. The mean serum concentration of MIA in these patients was 17.22 ng/ml, whereas in the 359 patients without metastasis, 6.74 ng/ml ($p < 0.001$). Sixteen of the 31 patients presented with metastatic disease during follow-up. These patients showed a MIA of 6.49 ng/ml before and of 17.44 ng/ml after the development of metastasis ($p = 0.001$). Comparing different apical tumor thickness to MIA serum concentrations in patients without metastasis, no significant correlation was found. A correlation between local therapy and MIA serum concentrations could neither be seen.

Conclusion: The statistically highly significant elevation of MIA serum levels in patients with metastatic disease from melanoma suggests a promising role as a serum marker for monitoring these patients.

In: Metastatic Melanoma
Editors: S.A. Klein and J.P. Beckler
ISBN 978-1-61209-915-6

Chapter I

Experimental Treatments for Blocking Melanoma Metastasis

***Marco Velasco-Velázquez*[*1,2], *Nidia Rodríguez-Rivera*[1], *Marisol de la Fuente-Granada*[3], *Vladimir Popov*[1] *and Mayra Pérez-Tapia*[3]**

[1]Departamento de Farmacología, Facultad de Medicina, Universidad Nacional Autónoma de México. México D.F., México

[2]Department of Cancer Biology, Thomas Jefferson University. Philadelphia, USA

[3]Departamento de Inmunología, Escuela Nacional de Ciencias Biológicas, Instituto Politécnico Nacional. México D.F., México

Abstract

The incidence and mortality rate of cutaneous melanoma have been increasing more rapidly than any other cancer over the last three decades.

* Corresponding author: Marco A. Velasco-Velázquez, Ph.D., Departamento de Farmacología, Facultad de Medicina, Universidad Nacional Autónoma de México. Apdo. Postal 70-297, Ciudad Universitaria, México D.F. 04510, México. Phone/Fax: +52-55-56232282. E-mail: marcovelasco@unam.mx.

The leading cause of mortality in melanoma patients is metastasis formation. Thus, it is necessary to find treatments that can block metastasis to improve survival of melanoma patients. The production of metastases is a highly complex process by which some melanoma cells move away from the primary tumor and colonize other organs. This process requires phenotypical changes that allow melanoma cells to migrate, survive in the blood circulation, extravasate, and proliferate in a tissue with a different microenvironment. Accordingly, new therapies aimed to block metastasis must target cellular functions like adhesion, migration, invasion, and homing. Having a different mechanism of action than cytotoxic and cytostatic drugs, such therapies could be used in combination with the current ones. This chapter reviews some key signaling pathways that affect melanoma metastasis and discusses the targeting of those pathways in different preclinical models. Such strategies may become the basis for the generation of new therapeutic alternatives for melanoma.

Introduction

Among the several different types of skin cancers in humans, basal cell carcinomas (BCCs), squamous cell carcinomas (SCCs), and melanomas represent the major group. BCCs do not proliferate rapidly and rarely metastasize, while SCCs are more malignant with a tendency of being highly metastatic. Melanomas are usually highly proliferative, invasive, and are most frequently metastatic. Melanoma accounts for nearly 4% of skin cancer cases but, because its highly metastatic capability, for 74% of all skin cancer mortalities [1]. Therefore, melanoma is one of the deadliest forms of cancer and its treatment continues to be challenging.

In contrast with other common cancer types, like breast and lung cancers, melanoma incidence has been rising over time. In US, more than 68,000 cases of melanoma were diagnosed during 2009 [2]. Given the high malignancy of melanoma, most of the patients develop metastasis, particularly to gastrointestinal tract, lungs, liver, brain and bones [3, 4]. Once the melanoma is invasive the 10-year survival rate for patients is less than 10% [5]. Available treatments for melanoma, either single-agent or combination chemotherapy, usually produce response rates ranging from 5 to 25% but do not improve survival rate [6]. Moreover, experimental evidence suggests that metastasis formation can be enhanced by treatment with cytotoxic drugs or radiotherapy [7]. These data emphasize the need for successful new therapies for metastatic melanoma. In this chapter we review and discuss some of the many therapeutic approaches currently under pre-clinical investigation for the development of metastatic melanoma.

The Metastatic Phenotype of Melanoma

Metastasis is a complex process involving many sequential steps. During the metastatic process, cancer cells invade the surrounding tissues and enter into the blood vessels. The cells that survive in the circulation can eventually arrest in the microvasculature and leave from blood by extravasation. Finally, the metastatic cells have to be able to respond to the local microenvironment in order to proliferate at distant organs [8]. The ability to invade and dissipate differs metastatic cells from noninvasive cancer cells. In melanomas, just like in other carcinomas, the difference between metastatic and non-metastatic outcome is due to several factors. Some genes have been pointed as crucial in the development of a metastatic phenotype.

The gene *nm23*, also known as NDP kinase, was first identified on K-1735 melanoma derived cell lines and was found to be poorly expressed on highly metastatic cells [9]. The metastasis suppressive activity of *nm23* has also been documented on other tumor types [10] and overexpression of the gene on highly metastatic cell lines decreased migration *in vitro* and metastasis *in vivo* [11]. It is likely that the fundamental cellular role of Nm23 is in differentiation and that this same role contributes to a lower metastatic threshold in cells that express this gene [12]. On MDA-MB-435 and MDA-MB-231 human breast carcinoma cells treated with dexamethasone or medroxyprogesterone acetate (MPA), protein levels of Nm23-H1 and Nm23-H2 proteins were increased and this resulted in the inhibition of migration *in vitro* without changing the cell proliferation [13]. Overexpression of Nm23 inMelJuSo human melanoma [14] and K-1735 TK murine melanoma cells [15] also resulted on metastasis reduction on mice models.

Other genes implicated on metastasis reduction are Breast Metastasis Suppressor 1 (BRMS1) and KISS1 [16]. BRMS1 mRNA expression was high in melanocytes but barely detectable in advanced/metastatic cell lines. BRMS1 overexpressing MelJuSo and C8161.9 human melanoma cell lines did not alter their tumorigenicity, but significantly suppressed their metastasis capability [17]. KISS1 gene produces kisspeptin, which binds to the G-protein coupled receptor GPR54 (also known as AXOR12 or hOT 7T 175). KISS1 expression was found in primary cultures of early melanomas, while it was lost in nearly half of the samples from large primary melanomas (>4 mm thickness) and metastases [18]. KISS1 maintains disseminated tumor cells in a dormant state after they have seeded other tissues [19]. In animal models, KISS1 expression blocked the ability of melanoma cancer cells to colonize and proliferate at secondary sites in cancer xenograft models [20]. On clinical trials, administration of kisspeptin-54, the protein encoded by KISS1, did not cause any reportable side effects. However, these treatments resulted in a robust release of gonadotropins [21], which is consistent with the finding that kisspeptin-54 stimulates the hypothalamic-pituitary-gonadal (HPG) axis in animal models and also plays an important role on human reproduction [22]. Thus, treatments that lead to an increase on the expression of metastasis-suppressor genes may constitute a translational strategy for the limitation of metastatic colonization in high risk cancer patients.

On the other hand, melanoma metastatic cells exhibit gain-of-function mutations that have been related to its malignancy. For example, B-RAF mutations are responsible, in large part, for the constitutive hyperactivation of survival/antiapoptotic pathways such as the MAPK, NF-κB, and PI3K/AKT in melanoma cells [23]. These pathways regulate the expression of genes like fibronectin, vimentin, several matrix metalloproteinases (MMPs), and the inhibition of E-cadherin, promoting epithelial-mesenchymal transition (EMT) [23]. The importance of B-RAF in melanoma biology and the fact that is also over-activated in other malignancies have lead to the development of several B-RAF inhibitors (reviewed by [24]). Sorafenib (BAY 43-9006) is a biaryl modified urea molecule that competes with ATP for binding RAF kinase inhibiting it [25]. Sorafenib also inhibits VEGF-R [26, 27], reducing tumor cell proliferation and angiogenesis. Sorafenib has been approved by the FDA for the treatment of advanced renal cell carcinoma [23]. In the case of melanoma, single sorafenib treatment has shown low toxicity and side effects retarding human melanoma growth and angiogenesis in mice by inhibition of MEK/ERK [27, 28] but showed no effect on lung metastasis [29]. The combination of sorafenib with the chemotherapeutic agents carboplatin and paclitaxel showed no significant difference on the overall survival of melanoma patients [30], suggesting that new treatments for the metastatic melanoma are still required.

Targets for the Development of Anti-Metastatic Therapies for Melanoma

Current systemic therapeutic approaches for melanoma are unsuccessful in part because the chemosensitivity of primary tumor and metastatic cells is different. The development of anti-metastatic therapies would increase the success rate of surgery and/or chemotherapy [8]. In order to block dissemination, therapies must target one of the steps of the metastatic cascade and not cell viability. Therefore, the cellular processes involved in metastasis as well as the molecules controlling those processes are obvious targets for the development of anti-metastatic drugs.

Cellular Motility and Invasiveness

Cancer cell invasiveness is one of the main requirements for metastasis. In order to gain access to new tissues, metastatic cells must interact with extracellular matrix (ECM) and activate migration-promoting pathways. The basic migration machinery involves at least three important categories of molecules: i) adhesion receptors and their ligands, ii) proteases, and iii) cytoskeletal proteins. All these components need to act in a coordinated manner in order to promote active migration. For example, integrin receptors activation produces both signaling that regulates the expression and secretion of proteases and actin-myosin contraction [31]. Changes on adhesion capability between cells and ECM have also been observed, mainly during intravasation/exavasation [32, 33]. As an outcome, several ECM-degrading enzymes have been reported to be altered on cancer metastasis, as matrix metalloproteinases, cathepsins, and urokinase plasminogen activator (u-PA) [34-37]. Also secretion of chemokines and growth factors by cancer or surrounding cells lead to the activation or over-expression of migration related signaling pathways like PI3K, Rac, Rho, ROCK or MLCK [38-43]. Pharmacological inhibitors that affect those basic components of migration machinery have been developed to interfere with metastasis.

Integrin Receptors

Integrins are evolutionary conserved cell adhesion receptors that play important roles on developmental and pathological process [44]. They are constituted by heterodimers that bind different molecules on ECM. The integrins generate signals from inside and outside the cell, representing the cellular link to the external environment [45]. Different integrin heterodimers have specialized functions on the maintenance or loss of the "normal" phenotype [46]; accordingly, integrins receptors are related with metastatic capability on melanomas and other cancers. For example $\alpha3\beta1$ integrin (VLA-3), a receptor for fibronectin, vitronectin, laminin, and kalinin/epiligrin, appears to be increased in malignant melanoma correlating with the degree of dermal invasiveness [47, 48]. On A375 melanoma cell line, $\alpha3\beta1$ integrin interaction with laminin-5 produced in the epidermis is involved in cell migration, invasion, and degradation of extracellular matrix proteins by induction of MMP-9 secretion [33]. Similarly, elevated levels of $\alpha2\beta1$ integrin (VLA-2) and $\alpha6\beta1$ integrin (VLA-6) are found in highly invasive and metastatic cell lines compared with normal cultured melanocytes and non-metastatic melanoma cell lines [46]. Highly metastatic cell lines also display an increased adhesion of the integrin ligands laminin and collagen [46, 49].

Melanoma metastasis can be blocked by targeting the different subunits of integrin receptors. The peptide sequence Arginine-Glycine-Aspartate (RGD) was first identified as the minimal structure recognized by cells in the large, adhesive glycoprotein fibronectin [50]. The RGD sequence is present in other ECM proteins that interact with adhesion receptors. For the integrin family, RGD sequence is recognized by 8 of the 24 integrin receptors. Some ECM molecules expose their RGD sequence upon denaturalization or cleavage allowing cells to bind these ligands [44]. The high affinity of some integrins for this sequence has been used as another approach for generating anti-metastatic drugs, developing molecular devices endowed with tumor-targeting functions and carrying cytotoxic components.

The first evidence that RGD sequence could work as anti-metastatic was shown by Humphries *et. al.* in 1986 when they co-injected the pentapeptide sequence Gly-Arg-Gly-Asp-Ser (GRGDS) with B16-F10 murine melanoma cells in C57BL/6 mice. They found a significant inhibition of lung metastasis that was dependent of the GRGDS dose [51]. Experiments with amino acid residue substitution showed that the core sequence responsible for cell recognition was Arg-Gly-Asp and that the surrounding amino acids were not essential [50].

The disintegrins are natural peptides that contain the RGD sequence. These peptides can also decrease the metastatic potential of cancer cells. Trigramin, a cysteine-rich, RGD-containing peptide isolated from the venom of the *Trimeresurus gramineus* snake inhibited the adhesion of human melanoma cells to fibrinogen and fibronectin [52]. Other cysteine-rich RGD-containing peptides were isolated from the venom of various vipers and are also potent inhibitors of both platelet aggregation and cell-substratum adhesion [53]. Albolabrin, isolated from the venom of *Trimeresurus albolabris*, inhibited the attachment of B16-F10 mouse melanoma cells to either fibronectin or laminin [54]. Triflavin, purified from *Trimeresurus flavoviridis* snake venom binds via its RGD sequence to $\alpha5\beta1$, $\alpha3\beta1$, and $\alpha v\beta3$ integrin receptors expressed on the surface of cancer cells, inhibiting B16-F10 cell adhesion to extracellular fibronectin and vitronectin [55]. The injection of four disintegrins: albolabrin, eristostatin, barbourin, and echistatin inhibited formation of experimental lung metastases in a murine model of melanoma [53].

Proteases

Changes on adhesion capability between cells and ECM have been observed, mainly during intravasation/exavasation [32, 33]. As outcome, several alterations on ECM-degrading enzymes have been reported on cancer metastasis. Metalloproteinases, cathepsins, and urokinase plasminogen activator (u-PA) [34-37] are important for the invasive capability of melanoma cells. Therefore, pharmacological inhibitors that block interactions of ECM and migration have been developed to interfere with metastasis.

Matrix metalloproteinases (MMPs) are a family of zinc-dependent neutral endopeptidases possessing the ability to degrade extracellular matrix components. MMPs degrade different structural components of the extracellular matrix and many other cell membrane and pericellular proteins, including cell membrane precursor forms of growth factors and others. Human MMP family is currently consisted of 23 members, which can further be divided into 8 subgroups depending on the substrate specificity [56, 57].

The activity of MMPs is specifically inhibited by tissue inhibitors of metalloproteinase and by nonspecific proteinase inhibitors. The presence of both, MMPs and their inhibitors, is essential in many physiological stages where the specific remodeling of the extracellular matrix is needed. However, since the extracellular matrix is hardly penetrable, presence of MMPs and their activity confers advantages in human carcinogenesis. Since the MMPs are crucial for metastatic melanomas, their function in the carcinogenesis has been investigated in depth. High serum levels of MMPs are associated with rapid progression in patients with metastatic melanomas [58].

Some of the anti-metastatic drugs that inhibit ECM-degrading enzymes are polyphenolic flavonoid compounds extracted from plants or fungus that had already been used on traditional medicine in the past. These pholyphenolic compounds have been reported to possess substantial skin photoprotective effects against solar ultraviolet (UV) radiation which has been implied in various skin diseases including melanoma and non-melanoma skin cancers [59]. In addition, they may have different effects on proliferation and survival pathways but the main mechanism involved in metastasis inhibition is the inactivation of MMPs and u-PA, which reduces the extravasation capacity of tumor cells.

Some polyphenolic flavonoid compounds, like silymarin and silibinin, do not completely inhibit ECM-degrading enzymes but reduce their expression importantly, which reduces metastasis significantly. Silymarin and silibinin are natural compounds isolated from milk thistle seed extracts (*Silybum marianum*). Silymarin is comprised of silibinin and its other stereoisomers, including isosilybin A, isosilybin B, silichristin, and silydianin. They have a potential anticancer activity inhibiting different steps on the whole cancer process including metastasis. The most commonly silymarin and silibinin products used on clinical trials are: Legalon, Thisilyn, Siliphos, and Silipide [60]. Preclinical studies have shown strong efficacy of silibinin to target cancer cell's migratory and invasive characteristics as well as their ability to metastasize to distant organs in hepatocellular carcinoma cells (HCC) [61]. In HCC cells, silibinin inhibited CDK2, CDK4, and CDC2 kinase activity, reduced the expression of MMP-2, MMP-9, and u-PA at a transcriptional level, and increased the abundance of the tissue inhibitor of MMP-2 (TIMP-2) on the translational or post-translational level [61]. All these molecules are involved in the regulation of EMT, which is a key step on initiating metastasis [62]. On SKH-1 hairless mice, silymarin inhibited UVB-induced skin tumor development in terms of incidence, multiplicity and growth [59]. Silibinin has been shown to inhibit photocarcinogenesis in mice when applied topically or in the diet via MAPK and Akt signaling inactivation [63]. In summary, silymarin and silibinin have an effect on proteases activation, adhesion, motility, and invasiveness as well as the supportive tumor-microenvironment components, thereby inhibiting metastasis [64].

A group from Taiwan showed that an ethanolic extract from *Terminalia catappa* (TCE) leaves contains flavonoid compounds with anti-metastatic activity. TCE extract inhibited the activities and protein levels of MMP-2, MMP-9, and u-PA on A549 and LLC cells *in vitro* and *in vivo* [65]. Four flavone compounds were responsible of the MMP-2 and u-PA inhibition: 7-

hydroxyflavanone, 5,6,7-trihydroxyflavanone, and 4′,5,7-trihydroxyflavanone [32]. In further studies, it was found that TCE may inhibit the phosphorylation of ERK1/2, JNK1/2, Akt, c-Jun, c-Fos and nuclear expression of NF-κB. EMSA assay with TCE revealed that the DNA-binding activity of AP-1 and NF-κB was also decreased [66].

Ruthenium complexes can also inhibit the release of MMPs. NAMI-A [(imH)[trans-RuCl4(dmso-S)(im)]; (im=imidazole, dmso=dimethylsulfoxide)] is a Ruthenium-(III) complex that has no effect on the primary tumor growth but a inhibited metastasis in MDA-MB-231 breast cancer cell lines [67] and displays reduced side effects on human trials [68]. NAMI-A reduces the release of MMP-2 and MMP-9 and increases the adhesion of KB and HeLa keratin-forming tumor cells at concentrations up to 100 times lower than those necessary to block cell cycle or to inhibit matrix metalloproteinase release for cell invasion. Cells treated with NAMI-A changed shape, with the extrusion of filopodia and of large lamellipodia, which increased their interactions with the substrate. This effect was attributed to stabilization, altered turnover, and sensitivity to cytochalasin D of actin filaments [69].

MMP inhibitors have been evaluated in clinical trials. For example, COL-3 is a potent inhibitor of MMP-2 and MMP-9 [70]. Phase I clinical studies using COL-3 showed disease stabilization in several patients who had a non epithelial type of malignancy, while the phototoxicity was dose-limiting [70]. However, even when a number of MMP inhibitors have gone through different phases of clinical trials none of these inhibitors has shown results that could ultimately be implemented as a standard therapy in treating melanomas as they have only had limited activity in patients with metastatic malignant melanomas [71].

The Actin Cytoskeleton

Actin polimerization is a reversible and highly dynamic process. By this intrinsic characteristic the actin cytoskeleton participates in cellular activities that require morphological changes. For example, the actin cytoskeleton plays key roles during cytokinesis, cell adhesion, and cell motility. In addition, it is involved in intracellular traffic regulation and in several signaling pathways, especially in those activated by adhesion and chemokine receptors [72].

The actin microfilaments are altered in transformed cells. Those changes, that involve alterations both in the actin organization and in microfilaments-regulating molecules, are directly related to the phenotypical changes displayed by invasive cancer cells [73]. Accordingly, the actin microfilaments have been pointed as therapeutic targets for metastasis inhibition [74].

Signaling Pathways That Control Actin Organization

The dynamic behavior of the actin cytoskeleton is space- and time-regulated by diverse signaling pathways. For example, binding of integrin adhesion receptors to their ligands produces the recruitment of several intracellular proteins that form focal adhesion complexes. Focal adhesions constitute important signaling centers that transduce signals that affect the actin cytoskeleton organization and regulate cellular processes like proliferation, survival or migration [75, 76]. In turn, changes in the actin cytoskeleton affect the function of adhesion receptors and can affect the adhesion receptor-mediated signaling [77].

Table1. Effect of 4-hydroxycoumarin (4-HC) on experimental metastasis

Treatment		Mice number	Metastatic incidence	Lung metastasis number/mouse	
	Control	9	100% (9/9)	53.8 ± 25.9	
In vitro	4-HC (500 μM)	9	100% (9/9)	8.8 ± 7.1	P<0.001
	Control	7	100% (7/7)	51.5 ± 20.9	
In vivo	4-HC (10 mg/Kg/day)	5	100% (5/5)	3.2 ± 2.2	P<0.01

Adapted from [85] and [89].

Thus, the molecules involved in the signal transduction that controls actin cytoskeleton rearrangements have been pointed as pharmacological targets for cancer treatment and metastasis inhibition [76, 78].

Paxillin is a multidomain adapter protein that participates in linking scaffolding and in signaling at focal adhesions [79]. The structural features of paxillin (reviewed by Brown and Turner [79] allow it to interact with different signaling proteins, such as FAK, Src, Crk, Csk, p120 RasGAP, and PTP-PEST [79, 80]. Thus, paxillin has been implicated in the regulation of diverse cellular events, including adhesion [81, 82], spreading [83], and motility [83, 84]. Our group has shown, in B16-F10 melanoma cells, that 4-hydroxycoumarin (4-HC) modifies the expression and activation of paxillin, impairing its relocalization to focal adhesions [85]. Thus, 4-HC reduces FAK and Rac1 activation [85]. Those effects alter the stability of the actin cytoskeleton, impairing the formation of stress fibers and lamellipodia and decreasing cell adhesion and of motility of B16-F10 cells [86].

4-HC also decreases the metastases formation in mouse models of melanoma. Both *in vitro* and *in vitro* treatments with 4-HC reduce the number of experimental lung metastasis caused by B16-F10 cells (Table 1). Even when other simple coumarins are cytotoxic or cytostatic to cancer cells [87], 4-HC does not alter cell viability, proliferation, nor long term cell survival of melanoma cells [85, 86, 88]. That information together with the fact that prophylactic administration of 4-HC is also effective in blocking experimental metastasis, lead us to the proposal that 4-HC may be affecting early steps of the metastatic cascade [85, 89]. However, 4-HC produces toxic effects in lung and kidney that would limit its use on clinical trials [89]. Nevertheless, 4-HC constitutes an example for the use of compounds that affect the expression of proteins important in the focal adhesion complex as anti-metastatic agents.

Mevalonate Pathway

The mevalonate pathway is important for the generation of isoprene moieties that provide the basis for the biosynthesis of molecules required for maintaining membrane integrity, steroid production, and cell respiration. It also allows the production of isoprene precursors for the prenylation of the Ras and Rho GTPases. The GTPases of Rho family participate actively in the dynamical changes of the actin cytoskeleton since they can modify the activity of actin-nucleating proteins, kinases, and phosphatases [90]. Thus, these GTPases play an important role on the regulation of cell proliferation, metastasis, and cell death on cancer therapies [91]. Statins and biophosphonates are inhibitors of the mevalonate pathway that have been used in clinics since many years in indications other than cancer [8]. As small GTPases are involved in all the modes of cancer cell motility, their inhibition can lead to an inhibition of metastasis. Thus, pharmacological inhibition of the mevalonate pathway has been seen as an alternative for cancer treatment. YM529/ONO-5920 a nitrogen-containing biophosphonate significantly inhibited lung metastasis, cell migration, invasion, and adhesion of B16-BL6 melanoma cells, as well as tumor metastasis and progression on hepatocellular carcinoma by suppressing the Rho/ROCK but no Ras pathway. It also showed no anti-proliferative effects primary tumor [92]. Pravastatin, fluvastatin and lovastatin reduced metastatic tumor formation of human pancreatic cancer to liver by inhibition of 3-hydroxy-3-methylglutaryl-coenzyme A (HMG-CoA)

[93]. Similarly, pravastatin reduced the lung metastasis of a rat hepatocellular carcinoma [94]. Nevertheless the specificity of inhibitors of the mevalonate pathway has yet to be well analyzed for compensatory effects between GTPases that may lead to non-desirable effects. For example, the Rac inhibitor NSC 23766 decreased migration of non-metastatic breast cancer cell lines MCF7 and T47D, but increased that of highly metastatic cells MDA-MB 231 and C3L5. This was probably mediated by the stimulation of RhoA as consequence of Rac1 downregulation [8].

Myosin Inhibitors

Myosin II is a key regulator for cell motility and adhesion. Myosin II activity is accelerated by phosphorylation of its regulatory light chain by myosin light chain kinase (MLCK). Suppression of MLCK has been used as an approach to inhibit motility and adhesion on different cancer cell lines [41]. KT5926, ML-7, and ML-9 MLCK inhibitors have shown a decrease in migration and adhesion of pancreatic cancer and glioma cells in a dose-dependent way [41, 95]. Thus, inhibition of MLCK could be a potential target for anti-metastatic therapies on melanoma.

Adhesion to Vascular Endothelium/Extravasation

Extravasation of tumor cells from capillary beds into the parenchyma of an organ is one of the steps of the metastatic cascade [96]. The key events during extravasation include tumor cell arrest or adhesion to the vasculature endothelium ("docking"), transition to more established cell contacts and numerous focal adhesions ("locking"), migration through the vasculature wall, adhesion to the subendothelial matrix and surrounding tissue, and subsequent remodeling of the target tissue stromal microenviroment [97].

The first steps of the extravasation process are similar to what is observed during leucocyte diapedesis [8]. In leukocytes, first, the endothelium, activated by cytokines produced in the local blood vessel after inflammation, expresses selectins, which act to 'dock' the leukocyte mucin-like cognate ligands to the endothelium. Then, this interaction mediates leukocyte tethering. Leukocyte rolling along endothelial cells in capillaries is activated by progressive interaction with a gradient of proinflammatory cytokines, which are secreted by endothelium activated by injury or infection. Leukocytes then arrest or "lock" to endothelium via juxtacrine activation of integrins on the surface of leukocytes which bind endothelial cell adhesion molecules (CAMs). CAMs are crucially involved in promoting cancer-endothelial cells interactions during extravasation [98]. Thus, anti-adhesion strategies are promising approaches for the development of new anti-metastatic therapies.

Selectins

Selectins are a family of transmembrane proteins containing an amino-terminal lectin domain for binding to ligands, an epidermal growth factor-like domain, 2-9 regulatory protein repeats, a transmembrane domain, and a short cytoplasmic tail [98]. This class of CAMs consists of three members, namely E-, L-, and P- selectins, which recognize several structures on tumor cell surfaces, leukocytes, platelets, and endothelial cells, thereby creating multiple binding possibilities [98]. Selectin ligand expression has been correlated with poor prognosis in carcinoma patients, indicating involvement of selectins in cancer progression. The presence of carcinoma cells expressing selectin ligands in blood circulation allows them to interact with selectins on platelets, leukocytes, and endothelial cells thereby leading to metastasis [99].

E- and P- selectins recognize sialylated fucosylated lactosaminoglycans, such as sialyl Lewis A (sLe^a) or sialyl Lewis X (sLe^x), which are normally expressed in the surface of various leukocyte subsets and promote leukocyte rolling on the cytokine-activated endothelial surface [100]. Normal human epidermal melanocytes (NHEM 685, neonatal) did not express sLe^x and poorly express sLe^a melanoma cells from tumor biopsies and human melanoma cell lines (M10-v, M24, and M101) expressed both sLe^x and sLe^a [101]. Not all melanoma cells express ligands for selectins [102, 103]; however, it has been shown that even melanoma cell lines that do not express sLe^x antigen can bound to E- or P-selectin [103,104].

In the absence of P-selectin melanoma cells expressing selectin ligands display reduced metastatic ability [105]. The absence of P-selectin led to a reduction of tumor seeding to the lung vasculature that was associated with a reduced platelet tumor cell emboli formation [106], showing that P-selectin-mediated tumor cell-platelet interactions are important for blood-borne metastasis. Similarly, attenuation of metastasis was observed in L-selectin deficient mice, strongly implicating leukocytes to be active facilitators of this process [107]. In the P- and L- selectin double deficient mice virtually no metastasis were observed, indicating a synergistic effect of both selectins during metastasis [108].

For the inhibition of selectin-mediated interactions, carbohydrate-based inhibitors of sLe^x biosynthesis have been developed. These agents consist of a per-acetylated disaccharide conjugated to a hydrophobic moiety. Peracetylation facilitates passive diffusion of the disaccharide across cell membranes, allowing entry into the Golgi, where sLe^x assembly takes place. The acetylated disaccharide undergoes deacetylation by endogenous esterases, which allows it to act as an intermediate in the biosynthesis of sLe^x. Assembly of oligosaccharides from the acetylated disaccharide inhibits the assembly of sLe^x from cellular glycoconjugates; thus, the per-acetylated disaccharide acts as an inhibitor of selectin-ligand formation [109]. The disaccharide per-*O*-acetylated GlcNAcβ1,3Galβ-*O*-naphthalenemethanol (AcGnG-NM) significantly inhibited spontaneous dissemination of B16-BL6 melanoma cells to the lungs from a primary s.c. tumor. However the number of treated animals was low and did not allow statistical conclusions [110]. Moreover different deoxygenated analogs of AcGnG-NM were described recently, one of this analogs blocks sLe^x formation and experimental tumor cell metastasis (Lewis Lung Carcinoma) without generation of oligosaccharide products [111].

A different strategy to block selectin-mediated adhesion has been the use of small molecules. IELLQAR peptide, which mimics selectin ligands, exhibits high binding to E-selectin. IELLQAR inhibited: i) the binding of sLe^x or sLe^a oligosaccharides to E-, P- and L-selectin; the adhesion of B16 melanoma cells expressing sLe^x (B16-FTIII cells) to E-selectin; and iii) the lung colonization by B16-FTIII melanoma cells [112].

Heparin is a complex mixture of natural glycosaminoglycans and contains a variety of biological activities (anticoagulant activity, inhibition of heparanase, antiangiogenic activity, among others). Heparin molecules are long unbranched polymers built of disaccharide repeats consisting of glucosamine an iduronic/galacturonic acid with a high degree of sulfatation [99]. Spontaneous and experimental metastasis can be effectively inhibited by heparin in different tumor models. Heparin was shown to bind to P- and L-selectin efficiently, despite the lack of obvious structural similarity to the natural selectin ligands such as $sLe^{x/a}$ [113, 114]. P-selectin-dependent melanoma cell-endothelial cell interactions *in vivo* are blocked by unfractionated heparin (UFH) treatment. UFH also inhibits experimental melanoma metastasis [105]. Most of the assays with heparin or its derivates have been done using single doses of heparin just before the injection of melanoma cells or right after, showing that the effect of heparins is in the initial steps of hematogenous metastasis formation.

Low-molecular-weight heparins (LMWHs) have been replacing UFH because of their advantages, such as predictable pharmacokinetics with increased bioavailability and half life time [115]. LMWHs as well as chemically modified heparins have been tested in experimental melanoma metastasis models. Nanoparin, a LMWH, inhibited the interactions of B16 melanoma cells with P-selectin-coated surfaces in a parallel flow chamber system. Nanoparin also decrease the number of experimental lung B16 melanoma metastasis [116]. Tinzaparin, a LMWH prepared from heparine by β-eliminative cleavage with heparinase [117], showed selectin inhibitory activity and attenuation of experimental lung metastasis on B16-F1 cells [118].

However the usefulness of heparin as an anticancer drug is limited by its modest therapeutic efficacy and the narrow therapeutic window due to its anticoagulant activity. The use of modified non-anticoagulant heparins has also showed an attenuation of metastasis on animal models, demonstrating that heparin anti-metastatic activity was independent from coagulation [119-122]. Multiple polyanionic heparinmimetics, which lack anticoagulant activity, have been tested as anticancer agents to identify compounds with a better efficacy and safety profile. LDH (LMWH-deoxycholic acid conjugate), produced by the covalent binding between the amine group of N-deoxycholyl-ethylenediamine (DOCA-NH2) and the carboxylic acids of heparin via amide linkage, is a chemical conjugate of LMWH and deoxycholic acid, with the advantage of be orally absorbable [123]. LDH attenuated metastasis experimentally induced by B16-F10 murine melanoma cells and its anti-metastatic activity was attributed to the interruption of the interactions between melanoma cells and activated platelets and between melanoma cells and human umbilical vascular endothelial cells by blocking selectin-mediated interactions [124].

Immunoglobilin Superfamily

The immunoglobulin CAMs (IgCAMs) are a large group of cell surface glycoproteins which contain an immunoglobulin like extracellular domain [98]. IgCAMs participate in adhesive interactions between tumor cells and the endothelium. The vascular cell adhesion molecule-1 (VCAM-1) is expressed on activated endothelium and is involved in the adhesion of white blood cells to the endothelium through interactions with integrins, such as the integrin α4β1 (VLA-4) [125]. Similarly, high-affinity interactions between integrin α4β1 and VCAM-1 accounted for the enhanced tumor extravasation mechanism [126]. VCAM-1 mediated vascular arrest of B16 melanoma cells at the metastatic sites depends on a cytokine cascade directly triggered by tumor cells, involving the sequential synthesis of TNF-α and IL-1β, and leading finally to the endothelial production of IL-18. Then, mature IL-18 induces VCAM-1, which facilitates the adhesion of tumor cell to endothelium [127, 128]. Both VCAM-1 and VLA-4 expressions have been reported to correlate with the metastatic pattern and clinical outcome in melanoma [129, 130].

Intercellular adhesion molecule-1 (ICAM-1, CD54) expressed on endothelial cells is one of the major cell surface glycoproteins that contribute to cell adhesion processes [131]. ICAM-1 expression has also been associated with metastatic potential of malignant melanoma cells [132]. TNF-α upregulates the activation of the transcription factor NF-κB [133], the expression of ICAM-1 [134, 135], integrin expression [136], and migration and invasion *in vitro* [137, 138] in a range of human melanoma cells.

IgCAMs as well as the proinflammatory cytokines that regulate their expression are possible therapeutic targets for metastatic melanoma. Since the counter-receptors for the IgCAMs belong to the integrin family, blocking peptides similar to those described under the section "*Integrins*" have been used to target IgCAM-mediated adhesion. Eristostatin has shown bind integrin α4β1, and inhibit melanoma cell adhesion to VCAM-1. Eristostatin inhibited adhesion of a highly metastatic human melanoma cell line (MV3) and α4-cDNA transfected CHO cells to VCAM-1, while adhesion to other ligands via other integrins was not affected [139].

Several flavonoids with anti-inflammatory activity have been proved to affect metastatic capability by reducing IgCAMs expression on the vascular endothelium. Apigenin (4',5,7-trihydroxyflavone) inhibited IL-1 and TNF-α-induced endothelial expression of ICAM-1 and VCAM [140, 141]. Apigenin inhibited polymorphonuclear leukocytes and peripheral blood lymphocytes adhesion to TNF-α stimulated HUVECs and blocked lung colonization of B16-BL6 melanoma cells [142]. Similarly, quercetin (3,3',4',5,7-pentahydroxy-flavone), a naturally occurring dietary flavonol, downregulated TNF-α-induced ICAM-1 expression. This effect is partially mediated by the inhibition of AP-1 transactivation induced by TNF-α [143]. Quercetin has also shown to inhibit lung colonization of B16-BL6 cells [142]. Pterostilbene (3,5-dimethoxy-4'-hydroxystilbene; PTER), a naturally occurring small polyphenol, inhibited metastatic growth of B16M-F10 cells in the liver, when administered in conjunct with quercetin. One of the mechanisms involved in this effect was the inhibition of VCAM-1 expression in the hepatic sinusoidal endothelium, which consequently decreases B16-F10 cell adhesion to the endothelial cells [144]. Finally, amentoflavone, which is the active polyphenolic component of *Biophytum sensitivum* and *Selaginella* species, significantly reduced tumor nodule formation using B16-F10 melanoma-induced experimental lung metastasis. Amentoflavone significantly decreased the serum levels of IL-1β, IL-6, TNF-α in metastasis induced animals. This compound inhibited the activation and nuclear translocation of p65, p50, c-Rel subunits of NF-κB [145]. Flavonoid inhibitory activity on the expression of endothelial adhesion molecules has been also observed in humans [146], suggesting that flavonoids may be useful for melanoma and other cancer types therapies.

MCAM, previously known as MUC18, Mel-CAM or CD146, is an IgCAM [147]. MCAM can mediate heterotypic adhesion between cells, although the counter receptor or ligand for MCAM has not yet been identified [148]. MCAM expression is associated with advanced and metastatic tumors, while its expression on tumors with low probability of metastasizing is less frequent [149]. There is a positive correlation between MCAM expression and the ability of human melanoma cell lines to metastasize in nude mice [150]. Overexpression of MUC18 in a low metastatic melanoma cell line, SB-2, causes an increase in tumorigenicity and metastatic potential in nude mice and increased attachment to human endothelial cells [151]. A fully humanized antibody directed against MUC18 (ABX-MA1) has been tested in murine melanoma models. The anti-metastatic effect of ABX-MA1 was determined by the administration of MUC18 positive melanoma cells (A375SM and WM2664) intravenously into nude mice to produce experimental lung metastases. The incidence and the number of lung metastases of both cell lines were lower in ABX-MA1 treated mice than in the controls [152]. ABX-MA1 inhibited the attachment of metastatic melanoma cells to HUVECs, affecting directly the extravasation step in the process of metastasis. ABX-MA1-treated tumors also exhibited a decrease in angiogenesis, suggesting that MUC18 is also important during the growth of new blood vessels into the secondary tumor.

Signals from the Metastatic Site

Once the cells gain access to blood circulation, they could potentially metastasize in any organ; however, this does not occur. Specific tissues exhibit characteristic that make them better sites for metastatic growth. Those target tissue must express signals that: i) attract cancer cells to them; ii) provide a favorable microenvironment to establish and proliferate; and iii) allow the neovascularization of the secondary tumor (reviewed in the next section). The need of all these characteristics for the development of macrometastasis has lead to the proposal of a pre-metastatic niche exist [153]. For example, it has been shown that micrometastasis can appear even 10 years prior the first clinically apparent macrometastasis [154]. Such evidence proves that if the microenvironment is not adequate, cancer cells can remain dormant after arriving to the target tissue.

Chemokines and their receptors have been shown to play a key role at the metastatic cascade. These molecules can direct chemotaxis and homing to specific organs, and are also involved in the creation of an adequate niche. Chemokines are soluble proteins of low molecular mass (5-15 kDa) [155] with chemoattractant activity that bind to an 18-member family of G protein-coupled receptors to mediate intracellular signaling. The physiologic function of these receptor/ligand pairs is to direct the migration of leukocytes, expressing a subset of receptors, to sites of tissue injury or inflammation. The expression of both, chemokines and chemokine receptors is strongly up-regulated during tumorigenesis. Metastatic melanoma cells express chemokine receptors that play a major role in specifying the organ site for metastasis, based upon receptor detection of the chemokine gradient elaborated by a specific organ/tissue [156].

Chemokines That Promote Homing

CXCR4 is a G protein-coupled receptor that binds CXCL12 (stromal-derived factor 1, SDF-1). The CXCR4/CXCL12 axis has been the most studied pathway in relation to the homing of metastasis cells [157-159]. The importance of CXCR4 expression in metastatic cancer was first described by Müller *et al.* They demonstrated that primary tumors of breast cancer express CXCR4 and that the inhibition of CXCR4 with blocking antibodies markedly decreased experimental lung metastases [158]. CXCR4 is also expressed in human melanoma cells lines (MeWo and A375) [157], primary melanomas, and melanoma liver and pulmonary metastases [160-163]. Expression of CXCR4 correlates with poor prognosis in patients with malignant melanoma and the percentage of melanoma cells that express CXCR4 correlates inversely with months of disease free survival [164]. Murakami *et al.* showed that a high expression of CXCR4 dramatically enhanced the metastatic accumulation of B16 melanoma cells in lungs [160]. On the other side knocking down CXCR4 in melanoma cells impairs melanoma metastasis to the lung in a murine xenograft model [165].

The ligand for CXCR4, CXCL12 is abundantly expressed in lung, lymph nodes, liver and bone marrow [166]. The CXCL12/CXCR4 axis is a key regulator of the tropism of melanoma cells to these organs [167]. CXCR4 antagonists have been developed and characterized for their therapeutic potential in HIV infection and inflammatory diseases. However, the evaluation of the anti-metastatic potential of these compounds is still on preclinical phases.

The small peptide T22, [Tyr-5,12,Lys-7] polyphemusin, a CXCR4 antagonist, was first described as an inhibitor of HIV-cell fusion, and was synthesized through modification of polyphemusin which is highly abundant in hemocyte debris of horseshoe crab (*Limulus polyphemus*) [168]. T22 blocks metastatic implantation into lungs of CXCR4-transduced B16 melanoma cells [160]. Smaller analogs of T22 retain the anti-metastatic activity. T140, a 14-residue peptide with a single disulfide bridge [169], inhibited the CXCL12 induced migration of human breast cancer cell lines and shown a significant reduction in pulmonary metastasis [170]. TN14003, which is a derivative of T140 [171], blocked migration and invasion of $CXCR4^+$ cells of pancreatic cancer [172] and decreased pulmonary metastasis in a breast cancer metastasis animal model [173]. 4F-benzoyl-TE14011, which is an analog based in T22 and T140, significantly reduced the number of pulmonary metastasis formed by B16-BL6 melanoma cells expressing CXCR4 after a single subcutaneous administration of this compound in biodegradable poly D,L-lactic acid (PLA) microcapsules [174]. An advantage of formulation based on biodegradable polymers such as PLA is the ability to maintain a relatively sustained drug release.

CTCE-9908, a 17-amino acid peptide, comprises a dimerized sequence of the disordered N-terminal region of SDF-1α, therefore it blocks the ligand binding to the CXCR4 receptor. CTCE-9908 shown a decrease in the number of lung metastasis when tested in the model of experimental metastasis with B16 murine melanoma cells that overexpressed human CXCR4 [175]. The bicyclam AMD3100 was the first non-peptide, small-molecule CXCR4 inhibitor reported in the literature [176]. Originally described as a highly potent and selective inhibitor of HIV-1 and HIV-2 replication [177], it blocks the CXCL2/CXCR4-axis in various cancers, affecting tumor growth as well as metastasis. AMD3100 inhibited invasion and metastasis activity of the colorectal cancer cell line SW480 [178], blocked the metastatic potential of HCT116 cells to form liver metastasis [179], and delayed the initial growth of experimentally produced lung metastases of 4T1 breast cancer cells [180]. Moreover, it has been seen that AMD3100 inhibits spontaneous and CXCL12-induced proliferation of melanoma cells [161].

CTCE-9908 is in a phase I/II trial indicated for solid tumors, meanwhile AMD3100 is in phase II/III indicated for multiple myeloma, acute myeloid leukemia and solid tumors. Even when these trials are not specifically directed to test metastatic melanoma, the successful results that these molecules could have may be relevant to metastatic melanoma, where the importance of CXCL2/CXCR4-axis has been proved.

CXCR3, which is the receptor for MIG (CXCL9), IP-10 (CXCL10), and CXCL11, has been associated with metastasis to lymph nodes [157, 181, 182]. CXCR3 has been detected in several melanoma cell lines, both murine (B16-F10) and human (BLM, SK-Mel 37) [157, 181]. It has also been detected in human primary cutaneous melanoma [182] and in samples from lymph-node melanoma metastasis [157]. Increased expression of CXCL9 and CXCL10 in the lymph nodes by complete Freund's adjuvant treatment facilitated homing of tumor cells to the inflamed node through CXCR3. Antisense RNA targeting CXCR3 inhibited metastasis of B16-F10 melanoma to lymph nodes but did not affect the number of melanoma lung metastases [181]. Thus, CXCR3/CXCL9-CXCL10 axis appears to play a role related to melanoma trafficking to lymph nodes but not to other secondary organs [181]. However, the CXCR3 antagonist AMG487, when administered systemically, inhibited experimental lung metastases of breast adenocarcinoma cells [183], colorectal cancer cells [184], and osteosarcoma cells [185]. This suggests that for other cancer types CXCR3 participates in multiple-site metastasis.

CCR9 has been described as a homing receptor for melanoma metastasis to the small bowel. CCL25, the ligand for CCR9 is highly expressed in small bowel and thymus. A study demonstrated that 102 out of 198 melanomas metastasize to the small bowel and 88 of 102 melanomas with small bowel metastasis expressed CCR9 [186]. CCR9 expression on melanoma carries a greater than 60% chance that there will be bowel metastasis [186]. A selective small-molecule antagonist of CCR9 (GSK-1605786) has been used as a treatment of Crohn's disease in a phase II/III trial and as a treatment for celiac disease in a phase II trial [187].

Signals from the Niche

In order to constitute a metastatic niche, the target tissue has to undergone cellular changes. These include the recruitment and clustering of hematopoietic progenitor cells (HPC) expressing vascular endothelial growth factor receptor-1 (VEGF-R1) and VLA-4 (integrin α4β1) [188]. CXCR4 expression on HPC also promote an increase on CXCL12 expression in a positive feed-back loop [189]. In addition, bone marrow cells or endothelial progenitor cells (EPC) are needed at the metastatic site. Those cells express VEGF-R2 and participate in the upregulation of fibronectin (ligand of VLA-4) that prepares the microenvironment for cancer cells anchorage and further neovascularization [153, 188, 190]. Once the metastatic cell has reached this microenvironment, deregulated interactions with the surrounding, consolidate the metastatic niche that favors their survival, proliferation and/or differentiation [191]. If the proliferation or neovascularizacion signals are not present in the microenvironment the metastatic cells remain dormant [192]. Therefore, blocking the crosstalk between tumor cells and the microenvironment at metastatic sites would inhibit the formation of clinically relevant metastases [191, 193, 194].

For example, malignant melanoma cells express CCR7 receptors for the lymphatic chemokine CCL21 [195, 196]. CCL21 secreted by lymphatic system, has been identified as a key regulatory molecule in the switch of dormancy to metastasis in melanoma and breast cancer cells. The CCL21-soluble inhibitor, Chemotrap-1, is a human chemokine-binding Fc fusion protein that reduced both lymphatic invasion and lymphatic metastasis growth of CCR7-expressing melanoma cells *in vivo* [197].

Neoangiogenesis

Tumor dormancy can last long periods of time, but can be finished by neovascularization signals on the metastatic tissues [194]. Blocking neoangiogenesis would lead to an inhibition on metastatic growth. Factors that promote neovascularization on primary tumor are also required on the metastasis niche for new tumor growth [198, 199]. One of the main factors involved on this process is VEGF, secreted by endothelial cells and HPC. On endothelial cells, VEGF-R2 interacts with the platelet-derived growth factor receptor beta (PDGF-Rβ) and the integrin αvβ3 on focal adhesions. This promotes increased cell proliferation and migration of cells when attached to vitronectin, a ligand of αvβ3 integrin [200]. Accordingly, anti-αvβ3 antibodies can inhibit the VEGF-induced phosphorylation of VEGF-R2 when endothelial cells are bound to vitronectin without disrupting cell adhesion [201]. Consequently, treatments with inhibitory antibodies or other compounds capable of interfere with the interaction of integrin and tyrosine kinase receptors like VEGF-R2 and PDGF-R could be useful for designing treatments to block neoangiogenesis and growth once the target tissue has been reached.

The RDG sequence (see section "*Integrins*") has also been used to design antibodies or peptidomimetics against αvβ3 and αvβ5 integrins expressed in the tumor-associated cells [202]. These receptors are particularly important for the migration and survival of endothelial cells during neoangiogenesis [203]. The mouse monoclonal antibody LM609 preferentially reacts with αvβ3 integrin and inhibits it [204]. LM609 blocks neoangiogenesis without affecting existing blood vessels [203, 205]. A humanized variant of LM609 named Vitaxin retained the properties of the mouse antibody [206] and has already been evaluated clinical trials for melanoma [207, 208], leiomyosarcoma [209], glioblastoma multiforme [208], and a group of patients with progressive tumors at stage IV disease [210]. In all cases some stabilization of the disease was reported with little or no toxicity.

Synthetic RGD peptidomimetics that inhibit αvβ3 and αvβ5 integrins have been tried on different epithelial cells and cancer models *in vivo* and *in vitro*. The RGD-peptidomimetic S247 has also a potent antiangiogenic activity. S247 blocks the proliferation of endothelial cells but not tumor cells [211]. Prolonged treatment of epithelial cells, human vascular smooth muscle cells, and human umbilical vein endothelial cells resulted on loss of cell attachment and caspase-8 activation that lead to apoptosis (anoikis) on a FAK and Akt independent way [212, 213]. On the other hand, S247 can also affect the invasiveness of cancer cells. S247 decreased migration of breast cancer cells as well as lung metastasis with no reduction in growth of primary tumors and only a slight reduction in tumor cells detected in circulating blood [214].

Another peptide ligand containing the RGD sequence also currently under clinical trials is the cyclic pentapeptide c[-RGDf(NMe)V-] or cilengitide [45, 202, 215]. Cilengitide displays a strong affinity and selectivity to αvβ3 integrin (IC50 = 0.6 nM), and blocks the integrin binding to ECM with inhibition of neovascularization *in vitro* and *in vivo* as well and inducing detachment and anoikis on gliomas [216-218]. Cilengitide is toxic to endothelial cells *in vitro* by inducing TNF-mediated PKB/Akt activation [219]. Cilengitide showed and increase the anti-tumor activity of chemotherapy and radiotherapy on melanoma [220] and non-small-cell lung cancer models [221] that has been observed also at clinical trials [222]. In combination with gemcitabine, cilengitide inhibited rapid growth of highly vascularized head and neck tumor [223], and it is now at phase III study in combination with radio- and chemotherapy [224].

On the other hand several compounds can antagonize the growth factors required for angiogenesis or inhibit their expression. Silymarine (previously discussed) has also an anti-neovascularization activity [60]. It has been shown in different studies that silymarine/silibinin inhibit endothelial cell growth and survival by apoptosis [225]. On human umbilical vein endothelial cells (HUVEC) silymarine inhibited tube formation in dose-dependent way [225] and decreased secreted VEGF without affecting the morphology of several cancer cell lines [225-228]. Silymarine also promoted anti-angiogenic effects on hepatocellular carcinoma by down-regulation of MMP2 and CD34 [229].

Table 2. Strategies for inhibition of melanoma metastasis

Step in metastatic cascade	Strategy	Examples
Cell motility and invasiveness	Block of integrin receptors	RGD peptidomimetics, disintegrins
	Block/reduce expression of proteases	Pholyphenolic flavonoids, NAMI-A, COL-3
	Target the actin cytoskeleton	4-HC, statins, biophosphanates, MLCK inhibitors
Adhesion to vascular endotelium/extravasation	Block/reduce expression of selectins on endothelial cells	Carbohydrate-based inhibitors, peptides.
	Block/reduce expression of IgCAMs on endothelial cells or their counter-receptors on melanoma cells	Anti-immflamatory flavonoids, anti-IgCAMs antibodies, disintegrins
Homing	Block chemokine/chemokine receptor axes	Anti-CXCR4 antibodies, Chemokine receptor antagonists, blocking peptides, anti-sense RNA
	Block signals from the niche	CCR7 blocking peptides
Neoangiogenesis	Block endothelial cell migration/proliferation	Anti-integrin antibodies, RGD peptidomimetics
Multi-steps	----	Heparin, sylimarine

All of these effects correlated with a decrease of microvessel and vascular density *in vitro* and *in vivo* [228, 230, 231].

Minodronate, a nitrogen-containing bisphosphonate, inhibited melanoma growth *in vitro* and improved survival in nude mice injected with human malignant G361 melanoma cells, by suppressing the VEGF expression, DNA synthesis, and tube formation on endothelial cells [232].

Conclusion

Tumor metastasis is the leading cause of death in melanoma patients. Therapeutic strategies that specifically diminish the metastatic ability of cancer cells may lead to the development of improved adjuvant therapies against melanoma. New therapies aimed to block metastasis must target adhesion, migration, invasion, and homing of cancer cells or cell migration and proliferation of endothelial cells (Table 2). Even when most of the strategies discussed here are on preclinical phases, they may become the basis for the generation of new therapeutic alternatives against melanoma.

References

[1] Parkin, DM; Bray, F; Ferlay, J; Pisani, P. Global cancer statistics, 2002. CA *Cancer J. Clin.*, 2005 55(2): 74-108.

[2] Horner, MJRL; Krapcho, M; Neyman, N; Aminou, R; Howlader, N; Altekruse, SF; Feuer, EJ; Huang, L; Mariotto, A; Miller, BA; Lewis, DR; Eisner, MP; Stinchcomb, DG; Edwards, BK. SEER Cancer Statistics Review, 1975-2006. Bethesda, MD, USA: National Cancer Institute; 2009.

[3] Barnholtz-Sloan, JS; Sloan, AE; Davis, FG; Vigneau, FD; Lai, P; Sawaya, RE. Incidence proportions of brain metastases in patients diagnosed (1973 to 2001) in the Metropolitan Detroit Cancer Surveillance System. J Clin Oncol, 2004 22(14): 2865-72.

[4] Barth, A; Wanek, LA; Morton, DL. Prognostic factors in 1,521 melanoma patients with distant metastases. *J. Am. Coll Surg.*, 1995 181(3): 193-201.

[5] Balch, CM; Buzaid, AC; Soong, SJ; Atkins, MB; Cascinelli, N; Coit, DG; Fleming, ID; Gershenwald, JE; Houghton, A, Jr.; Kirkwood, JM;

McMasters, KM; Mihm, MF; Morton, DL; Reintgen, DS; Ross, MI; Sober, A; Thompson, JA; Thompson, JF. Final version of the American Joint Committee on Cancer staging system for cutaneous melanoma. *J. Clin. Oncol.*, 2001 19(16): 3635-48.

[6] Bhatia, S; Tykodi, SS; Thompson, JA. Treatment of metastatic melanoma: an overview. Oncology (Williston Park), 2009 23(6): 488-96.

[7] McMillan, TJ; Hart, IR. Enhanced experimental metastatic capacity of a murine melanoma following pre-treatment with anticancer drugs. *Clin. Exp. Metastasis*, 1986 4(4): 285-92.

[8] Perret, GY; Crepin, M. New pharmacological strategies against metastatic spread. *Fundam Clin. Pharmacol.*, 2008 22(5): 465-92.

[9] Lombardi, D. Commentary: nm23, a metastasis suppressor gene with a tumor suppressor gene aptitude? *J. Bioenerg. Biomembr.*, 2006 38(3-4): 177-80.

[10] Hartsough, MT; Steeg, PS. Nm23/nucleoside diphosphate kinase in human cancers. *J. Bioenerg. Biomembr.*, 2000 32(3): 301-8.

[11] Salerno, M; Ouatas, T; Palmieri, D; Steeg, PS. Inhibition of signal transduction by the nm23 metastasis suppressor: possible mechanisms. *Clin. Exp. Metastasis*, 2003 20(1): 3-10.

[12] Steeg, PS. Perspectives on classic article: metastasis suppressor genes. *J. Natl. Cancer Inst.*, 2004 96(6): E4.

[13] Ouatas, T; Halverson, D; Steeg, PS. Dexamethasone and medroxyprogesterone acetate elevate Nm23-H1 metastasis suppressor gene expression in metastatic human breast carcinoma cells: new uses for old compounds. *Clin. Cancer Res.*, 2003 9(10 Pt 1): 3763-72.

[14] Miele, ME; De La Rosa, A; Lee, JH; Hicks, DJ; Dennis, JU; Steeg, PS; Welch, DR. Suppression of human melanoma metastasis following introduction of chromosome 6 is independent of NME1 (Nm23). *Clin. Exp. Metastasis*, 1997 15(3): 259-65.

[15] Leone, A; Flatow, U; King, CR; Sandeen, MA; Margulies, IM; Liotta, LA; Steeg, PS. Reduced tumor incidence, metastatic potential, and cytokine responsiveness of nm23-transfected melanoma cells. *Cell,* 1991 65(1): 25-35.

[16] Steeg, PS; Ouatas, T; Halverson, D; Palmieri, D; Salerno, M. Metastasis suppressor genes: basic biology and potential clinical use. *Clin Breast Cancer*, 2003 4(1): 51-62.

[17] Shevde, LA; Samant, RS; Goldberg, SF; Sikaneta, T; Alessandrini, A; Donahue, HJ; Mauger, DT; Welch, DR. Suppression of human

melanoma metastasis by the metastasis suppressor gene, BRMS1. *Exp. Cell Res.*, 2002 273(2): 229-39.

[18] Debies, MT; Welch, DR. Genetic basis of human breast cancer metastasis. *J. Mammary Gland Biol. Neoplasia*, 2001 6(4): 441-51.

[19] Beck, BH; Welch, DR. The KISS1 metastasis suppressor: a good night kiss for disseminated cancer cells. *Eur. J. Cancer*, 2010 46(7): 1283-9.

[20] Lee, JH; Miele, ME; Hicks, DJ; Phillips, KK; Trent, JM; Weissman, BE; Welch, DR. KiSS-1, a novel human malignant melanoma metastasis-suppressor gene. *J. Natl. Cancer Inst.*, 1996 88(23): 1731-7.

[21] Dhillo, WS; Chaudhri, OB; Thompson, EL; Murphy, KG; Patterson, M; Ramachandran, R; Nijher, GK; Amber, V; Kokkinos, A; Donaldson, M; Ghatei, MA; Bloom, SR. Kisspeptin-54 stimulates gonadotropin release most potently during the preovulatory phase of the menstrual cycle in women. *J. Clin. Endocrinol. Metab.*, 2007 92(10): 3958-66.

[22] Dhillo, WS; Murphy, KG; Bloom, SR. The neuroendocrine physiology of kisspeptin in the human. *Rev. Endocr. Metab. Disord,* 2007 8(1): 41-6.

[23] Lin, K; Baritaki, S; Militello, L; Malaponte, G; Bevelacqua, Y; Bonavida, B. The Role of B-RAF Mutations in Melanoma and the Induction of EMT via Dysregulation of the NF-kappaB/Snail/RKIP/PTEN Circuit. *Genes Cancer*, 2010 1(5): 409-420.

[24] Wong, KK. Recent developments in anti-cancer agents targeting the Ras/Raf/ MEK/ERK pathway. *Recent. Pat. Anticancer Drug Discov.*, 2009 4(1): 28-35.

[25] Wellbrock, C; Hurlstone, A. BRAF as therapeutic target in melanoma. *Biochem Pharmacol*, 2010 80(5): 561-7.

[26] Egberts, F; Kahler, KC; Livingstone, E; Hauschild, A. Metastatic melanoma: scientific rationale for sorafenib treatment and clinical results. *Onkologie*, 2008 31(7): 398-403.

[27] Wilhelm, SM; Carter, C; Tang, L; Wilkie, D; McNabola, A; Rong, H; Chen, C; Zhang, X; Vincent, P; McHugh, M; Cao, Y; Shujath, J; Gawlak, S; Eveleigh, D; Rowley, B; Liu, L; Adnane, L; Lynch, M; Auclair, D; Taylor, I; Gedrich, R; Voznesensky, A; Riedl, B; Post, LE; Bollag, G; Trail, PA. BAY 43-9006 exhibits broad spectrum oral antitumor activity and targets the RAF/MEK/ERK pathway and receptor tyrosine kinases involved in tumor progression and angiogenesis. *Cancer Res.*, 2004 64(19): 7099-109.

[28] Karasarides, M; Chiloeches, A; Hayward, R; Niculescu-Duvaz, D; Scanlon, I; Friedlos, F; Ogilvie, L; Hedley, D; Martin, J; Marshall, CJ;

Springer, CJ; Marais, R. B-RAF is a therapeutic target in melanoma. *Oncogene*, 2004 23(37): 6292-8.

[29] Sharma, A; Tran, MA; Liang, S; Sharma, AK; Amin, S; Smith, CD; Dong, C; Robertson, GP. Targeting mitogen-activated protein kinase/extracellular signal-regulated kinase kinase in the mutant (V600E) B-Raf signaling cascade effectively inhibits melanoma lung metastases. *Cancer Res.*, 2006 66(16): 8200-9.

[30] Flaherty, KT; Schiller, J; Schuchter, LM; Liu, G; Tuveson, DA; Redlinger, M; Lathia, C; Xia, C; Petrenciuc, O; Hingorani, SR; Jacobetz, MA; Van Belle, PA; Elder, D; Brose, MS; Weber, BL; Albertini, MR; O'Dwyer, PJ. A phase I trial of the oral, multikinase inhibitor sorafenib in combination with carboplatin and paclitaxel. Clin. *Cancer Res.*, 2008 14(15): 4836-42.

[31] Friedl, P; Wolf, K. Tumour-cell invasion and migration: diversity and escape mechanisms. *Nat. Rev. Cancer*, 2003 3(5): 362-74.

[32] Yang, SF; Yang, WE; Kuo, WH; Chang, HR; Chu, SC; Hsieh, YS. Antimetastatic potentials of flavones on oral cancer cell via an inhibition of matrix-degrading proteases. *Arch. Oral. Biol.*, 2008 53(3): 287-94.

[33] Tsuji, T; Kawada, Y; Kai-Murozono, M; Komatsu, S; Han, SA; Takeuchi, K; Mizushima, H; Miyazaki, K; Irimura, T. Regulation of melanoma cell migration and invasion by laminin-5 and alpha3beta1 integrin (VLA-3). *Clin. Exp. Metastasis*, 2002 19(2): 127-34.

[34] Yoon, SO; Park, SJ; Yun, CH; Chung, AS. Roles of matrix metalloproteinases in tumor metastasis and angiogenesis. *J. Biochem. Mol. Biol.*, 2003 36(1): 128-37.

[35] Westermarck, J; Kahari, VM. Regulation of matrix metalloproteinase expression in tumor invasion. *FASEB J.*, 1999 13(8): 781-92.

[36] Yang, SF; Hsieh, YS; Lin, CL; Hsu, NY; Chiou, HL; Chou, FP; Chu, SC. Increased plasma levels of urokinase plasminogen activator and matrix metalloproteinase-9 in nonsmall cell lung cancer patients. *Clin. Chim. Acta.*, 2005 354(1-2): 91-9.

[37] Sameni, M; Dosescu, J; Sloane, BF. Imaging proteolysis by living human glioma cells. *Biol. Chem.*, 2001 382(5): 785-8.

[38] Allman, R; Cowburn, P; Mason, M. In vitro and in vivo effects of a cyclic peptide with affinity for the alpha(nu)beta3 integrin in human melanoma cells. *Eur. J. Cancer*, 2000 36(3): 410-22.

[39] Clark, EA; Golub, TR; Lander, ES; Hynes, RO. Genomic analysis of metastasis reveals an essential role for RhoC. *Nature*, 2000 406(6795): 532-5.

[40] Alper, O; Bergmann-Leitner, ES; Bennett, TA; Hacker, NF; Stromberg, K; Stetler-Stevenson, WG. Epidermal growth factor receptor signaling and the invasive phenotype of ovarian carcinoma cells. *J. Natl. Cancer Inst.,* 2001 93(18): 1375-84.

[41] Kaneko, K; Satoh, K; Masamune, A; Satoh, A; Shimosegawa, T. Myosin light chain kinase inhibitors can block invasion and adhesion of human pancreatic cancer cell lines. *Pancreas*, 2002 24(1): 34-41.

[42] Tsutsumi, S; Gupta, SK; Hogan, V; Collard, JG; Raz, A. Activation of small GTPase Rho is required for autocrine motility factor signaling. *Cancer Res.*, 2002 62(15): 4484-90.

[43] Somlyo, AV; Phelps, C; Dipierro, C; Eto, M; Read, P; Barrett, M; Gibson, JJ; Burnitz, MC; Myers, C; Somlyo, AP. Rho kinase and matrix metalloproteinase inhibitors cooperate to inhibit angiogenesis and growth of human prostate cancer xenotransplants. *FASEB J.,* 2003 17(2): 223-34.

[44] Barczyk, M; Carracedo, S; Gullberg, D. Integrins. *Cell Tissue Res.,* 2009 339(1): 269-80.

[45] Paolillo, M; Russo, MA; Serra, M; Colombo, L; Schinelli, S. Small molecule integrin antagonists in cancer therapy. *Mini. Rev. Med. Chem.*, 2009 9(12): 1439-46.

[46] Melchiori, A; Mortarini, R; Carlone, S; Marchisio, PC; Anichini, A; Noonan, DM; Albini, A. The alpha 3 beta 1 integrin is involved in melanoma cell migration and invasion. *Exp. Cell Res.*, 1995 219(1): 233-42.

[47] Weitzman, JB; Pasqualini, R; Takada, Y; Hemler, ME. The function and distinctive regulation of the integrin VLA-3 in cell adhesion, spreading, and homotypic cell aggregation. *J. Biol. Chem.*, 1993 268(12): 8651-7.

[48] Rousselle, P; Aumailley, M. Kalinin is more efficient than laminin in promoting adhesion of primary keratinocytes and some other epithelial cells and has a different requirement for integrin receptors. *J. Cell Biol.*, 1994 125(1): 205-14.

[49] Giannelli, G; Bergamini, C; Fransvea, E; Marinosci, F; Quaranta, V; Antonaci, S. Human hepatocellular carcinoma (HCC) cells require both alpha3beta1 integrin and matrix metalloproteinases activity for migration and invasion. *Lab. Invest.*, 2001 81(4): 613-27.

[50] Pierschbacher, MD; Ruoslahti, E. Variants of the cell recognition site of fibronectin that retain attachment-promoting activity. *Proc. Natl. Acad. Sci. USA*, 1984 81(19): 5985-8.

[51] Humphries, MJ; Olden, K; Yamada, KM. A synthetic peptide from fibronectin inhibits experimental metastasis of murine melanoma cells. *Science,* 1986 233(4762): 467-70.

[52] Knudsen, KA; Tuszynski, GP; Huang, TF; Niewiarowski, S. Trigramin, an RGD-containing peptide from snake venom, inhibits cell-substratum adhesion of human melanoma cells. *Exp. Cell Res.*, 1988 179(1): 42-9.

[53] Beviglia, L; Stewart, GJ; Niewiarowski, S. Effect of four disintegrins on the adhesive and metastatic properties of B16F10 melanoma cells in a murine model. *Oncol. Res.,* 1995 7(1): 7-20.

[54] Soszka, T; Knudsen, KA; Beviglia, L; Rossi, C; Poggi, A; Niewiarowski, S. Inhibition of murine melanoma cell-matrix adhesion and experimental metastasis by albolabrin, an RGD-containing peptide isolated from the venom of Trimeresurus albolabris. *Exp. Cell Res.*, 1991 196(1): 6-12.

[55] Sheu, JR; Huang, TF. Triflavin, an Arg-Gly-Asp-Containing Peptide, Inhibits B16-F10 Mouse Melanoma Cell Adhesion to Matrix Proteins via Direct Binding to Tumor Cells. *J. Biomed. Sci.*, 1996 3(5): 359-364.

[56] Coussens, LM; Fingleton, B; Matrisian, LM. Matrix metalloproteinase inhibitors and cancer: trials and tribulations. *Science,* 2002 295(5564): 2387-92.

[57] Egeblad, M; Werb, Z. New functions for the matrix metalloproteinases in cancer progression. *Nat. Rev. Cancer*, 2002 2(3): 161-74.

[58] Nikkola, J; Vihinen, P; Vuoristo, MS; Kellokumpu-Lehtinen, P; Kahari, VM; Pyrhonen, S. High serum levels of matrix metalloproteinase-9 and matrix metalloproteinase-1 are associated with rapid progression in patients with metastatic melanoma. *Clin. Cancer Res.*, 2005 11(14): 5158-66.

[59] Nichols, JA; Katiyar, SK. Skin photoprotection by natural polyphenols: anti-inflammatory, antioxidant and DNA repair mechanisms. *Arch. Dermatol. Res.*, 2010 302(2): 71-83.

[60] Ramasamy, K; Agarwal, R. Multitargeted therapy of cancer by silymarin. *Cancer Lett.,* 2008 269(2): 352-62.

[61] Varghese, L; Agarwal, C; Tyagi, A; Singh, RP; Agarwal, R. Silibinin efficacy against human hepatocellular carcinoma. *Clin. Cancer Res.*, 2005 11(23): 8441-8.

[62] Hsieh, YS; Chu, SC; Yang, SF; Chen, PN; Liu, YC; Lu, KH. Silibinin suppresses human osteosarcoma MG-63 cell invasion by inhibiting the ERK-dependent c-Jun/AP-1 induction of MMP-2. *Carcinogenesis,* 2007 28(5): 977-87.

[63] Mallikarjuna, G; Dhanalakshmi, S; Singh, RP; Agarwal, C; Agarwal, R. Silibinin protects against photocarcinogenesis via modulation of cell cycle regulators, mitogen-activated protein kinases, and Akt signaling. *Cancer Res.*, 2004 64(17): 6349-56.

[64] Deep, G; Agarwal, R. Antimetastatic efficacy of silibinin: molecular mechanisms and therapeutic potential against cancer. *Cancer Metastasis Rev.*, 2010 29(3): 447-63.

[65] Chu, SC; Yang, SF; Liu, SJ; Kuo, WH; Chang, YZ; Hsieh, YS. In vitro and in vivo antimetastatic effects of Terminalia catappa L. leaves on lung cancer cells. *Food Chem. Toxicol.,* 2007 45(7): 1194-201.

[66] Yang, SF; Chen, MK; Hsieh, YS; Yang, JS; Zavras, AI; Hsieh, YH; Su, SC; Kao, TY; Chen, PN; Chu, SC. Antimetastatic effects of Terminalia catappa L. on oral cancer via a down-regulation of metastasis-associated proteases. *Food Chem. Toxicol.*, 2010 48(4): 1052-8.

[67] Bergamo, A; Masi, A; Jakupec, MA; Keppler, BK; Sava, G. Inhibitory Effects of the Ruthenium Complex KP1019 in Models of Mammary Cancer Cell Migration and Invasion. *Met Based Drugs*, 2009 2009: 681270.

[68] Bergamo, A; Sava, G. Ruthenium complexes can target determinants of tumour malignancy. *Dalton Trans.*, 2007(13): 1267-72.

[69] Sava, G; Frausin, F; Cocchietto, M; Vita, F; Podda, E; Spessotto, P; Furlani, A; Scarcia, V; Zabucchi, G. Actin-dependent tumour cell adhesion after short-term exposure to the antimetastasis ruthenium complex NAMI-A. *Eur. J. Cancer*, 2004 40(9): 1383-96.

[70] Rudek, MA; Figg, WD; Dyer, V; Dahut, W; Turner, ML; Steinberg, SM; Liewehr, DJ; Kohler, DR; Pluda, JM; Reed, E. Phase I clinical trial of oral COL-3, a matrix metalloproteinase inhibitor, in patients with refractory metastatic cancer. *J. Clin. Oncol.,* 2001 19(2): 584-92.

[71] Quirt, I; Bodurth, A; Lohmann, R; Rusthoven, J; Belanger, K; Young, V; Wainman, N; Stewar, W; Eisenhauer, E. Phase II study of marimastat (BB-2516) in malignant melanoma: a clinical and tumor biopsy study of the National Cancer Institute of Canada Clinical Trials Group. *Invest. New Drugs*, 2002 20(4): 431-7.

[72] Barkalow, K; Hartwig, JH. Actin cytoskeleton. Setting the pace of cell movement. *Curr. Biol.*, 1995 5(9): 1000-2.

[73] Pawlak, G; Helfman, DM. Cytoskeletal changes in cell transformation and tumorigenesis. *Curr. Opin. Genet. Dev.,* 2001 11(1): 41-7.

[74] Jordan, MA; Wilson, L. Microtubules and actin filaments: dynamic targets for cancer chemotherapy. *Curr. Opin. Cell Biol.*, 1998 10(1): 123-30.

[75] Geiger, B; Bershadsky, A; Pankov, R; Yamada, KM. Transmembrane crosstalk between the extracellular matrix--cytoskeleton crosstalk. *Nat. Rev. Mol. Cell Biol.,* 2001 2(11): 793-805.

[76] Velasco-Velazquez, MA; Molina-Guarneros, JA; Mendoza-Patino, N; Sullivan Lopez, J; Mandoki, JJ. [Integrins and integrin-associated molecules: targets for the development of antimetastatic therapies]. *Rev. Invest Clin.*, 1999 51(3): 183-93.

[77] Schoenwaelder, SM; Burridge, K. Bidirectional signaling between the cytoskeleton and integrins. *Curr. Opin. Cell Biol.*, 1999 11(2): 274-86.

[78] Ruoslahti, E. Integrins as signaling molecules and targets for tumor therapy. *Kidney Int.,* 1997 51(5): 1413-7.

[79] Brown, MC; Turner, CE. Paxillin: adapting to change. *Physiol. Rev.*, 2004 84(4): 1315-39.

[80] Wang, Y; Gilmore, TD. Zyxin and paxillin proteins: focal adhesion plaque LIM domain proteins go nuclear. *Biochim. Biophys. Acta*, 2003 1593(2-3): 115-20.

[81] Sanders, MA; Basson, MD. Collagen IV-dependent ERK activation in human Caco-2 intestinal epithelial cells requires focal adhesion kinase. *J. Biol. Chem.*, 2000 275(48): 38040-7.

[82] Burridge, K; Turner, CE; Romer, LH. Tyrosine phosphorylation of paxillin and pp125FAK accompanies cell adhesion to extracellular matrix: a role in cytoskeletal assembly. *J. Cell Biol.*, 1992 119(4): 893-903.

[83] Jamieson, JS; Tumbarello, DA; Halle, M; Brown, MC; Tremblay, ML; Turner, CE. Paxillin is essential for PTP-PEST-dependent regulation of cell spreading and motility: a role for paxillin kinase linker. *J. Cell Sci.*, 2005 118(Pt 24): 5835-47.

[84] Petit, V; Boyer, B; Lentz, D; Turner, CE; Thiery, JP; Valles, AM. Phosphorylation of tyrosine residues 31 and 118 on paxillin regulates cell migration through an association with CRK in NBT-II cells. *J. Cell Biol.*, 2000 148(5): 957-70.

[85] Velasco-Velazquez, MA; Salinas-Jazmin, N; Mendoza-Patino, N; Mandoki, JJ. Reduced paxillin expression contributes to the antimetastatic effect of 4-hydroxycoumarin on B16-F10 melanoma cells. *Cancer Cell Int.*, 2008 8: 8.

[86] Velasco-Velazquez, MA; Agramonte-Hevia, J; Barrera, D; Jimenez-Orozco, A; Garcia-Mondragon, MJ; Mendoza-Patino, N; Landa, A; Mandoki, J. 4-Hydroxycoumarin disorganizes the actin cytoskeleton in B16-F10 melanoma cells but not in B82 fibroblasts, decreasing their adhesion to extracellular matrix proteins and motility. *Cancer Lett.*, 2003 198(2): 179-86.

[87] Lacy, A; O'Kennedy, R. Studies on coumarins and coumarin-related compounds to determine their therapeutic role in the treatment of cancer. *Curr. Pharm. Des.*, 2004 10(30): 3797-811.

[88] Kawaii, S; Tomono, Y; Ogawa, K; Sugiura, M; Yano, M; Yoshizawa, Y. The antiproliferative effect of coumarins on several cancer cell lines. *Anticancer Res.*, 2001 21(2A): 917-23.

[89] Salinas-Jazmin, N; de la Fuente, M; Jaimez, R; Perez-Tapia, M; Perez-Torres, A; Velasco-Velazquez, MA. Antimetastatic, antineoplastic, and toxic effects of 4-hydroxycoumarin in a preclinical mouse melanoma model. *Cancer Chemother Pharmacol.,* 2010 65(5): 931-40.

[90] Heasman, SJ; Ridley, AJ. Mammalian Rho GTPases: new insights into their functions from in vivo studies. *Nat. Rev. Mol. Cell Biol.*, 2008 9(9): 690-701.

[91] Fritz, G. Targeting the mevalonate pathway for improved anticancer therapy. *Curr. Cancer Drug Targets*, 2009 9(5): 626-38.

[92] Tanimori, Y; Tsubaki, M; Yamazoe, Y; Satou, T; Itoh, T; Kidera, Y; Yanae, M; Yamamoto, C; Kaneko, J; Nishida, S. Nitrogen-containing bisphosphonate, YM529/ONO-5920, inhibits tumor metastasis in mouse melanoma through suppression of the Rho/ROCK pathway. *Clin. Exp. Metastasis*, 2010.

[93] Kusama, T; Mukai, M; Iwasaki, T; Tatsuta, M; Matsumoto, Y; Akedo, H; Inoue, M; Nakamura, H. 3-hydroxy-3-methylglutaryl-coenzyme a reductase inhibitors reduce human pancreatic cancer cell invasion and metastasis. *Gastroenterology,* 2002 122(2): 308-17.

[94] Taras, D; Blanc, JF; Rullier, A; Dugot-Senant, N; Laurendeau, I; Vidaud, M; Rosenbaum, J. Pravastatin reduces lung metastasis of rat hepatocellular carcinoma via a coordinated decrease of MMP expression and activity. *J. Hepatol.*, 2007 46(1): 69-76.

[95] Gillespie, GY; Soroceanu, L; Manning, TJ, Jr.; Gladson, CL; Rosenfeld, SS. Glioma migration can be blocked by nontoxic inhibitors of myosin II. *Cancer Res.*, 1999 59(9): 2076-82.

[96] Nguyen, DX; Bos, PD; Massague, J. Metastasis: from dissemination to organ-specific colonization. *Nat. Rev. Cancer*, 2009 9(4): 274-84.

[97] Miles, FL; Pruitt, FL; van Golen, KL; Cooper, CR. Stepping out of the flow: capillary extravasation in cancer metastasis. *Clin. Exp. Metastasis*, 2008 25(4): 305-24.

[98] Makrilia, N; Kollias, A; Manolopoulos, L; Syrigos, K. Cell adhesion molecules: role and clinical significance in cancer. *Cancer Invest, 2009* 27(10): 1023-37.

[99] Borsig, L. Heparin as an inhibitor of cancer progression. *Prog. Mol. Biol. Transl. Sci.,* 2010 93: 335-49.

[100] Biancone, L; Araki, M; Araki, K; Vassalli, P; Stamenkovic, I. Redirection of tumor metastasis by expression of E-selectin in vivo. *J. Exp. Med.*, 1996 183(2): 581-7.

[101] Ravindranath, MH; Amiri, AA; Bauer, PM; Kelley, MC; Essner, R; Morton, DL. Endothelial-selectin ligands sialyl Lewis(x) and sialyl Lewis(a) are differentiation antigens immunogenic in human melanoma. *Cancer*, 1997 79(9): 1686-97.

[102] Miller, N; Vile, RG; Hart, IR. Selectin ligands on human melanoma cells. *Glycoconj J.,* 1996 13(1): 33-43.

[103] Kunzendorf, U; Kruger-Krasagakes, S; Notter, M; Hock, H; Walz, G; Diamantstein, T. A sialyl-Le(x)-negative melanoma cell line binds to E-selectin but not to P-selectin. *Cancer Res.*, 1994 54(4): 1109-12.

[104] Kaytes, PS; Geng, JG. P-selectin mediates adhesion of the human melanoma cell line NKI-4: identification of glycoprotein ligands. *Biochemistry*, 1998 37(29): 10514-21.

[105] Ludwig, RJ; Boehme, B; Podda, M; Henschler, R; Jager, E; Tandi, C; Boehncke, WH; Zollner, TM; Kaufmann, R; Gille, J. Endothelial P-selectin as a target of heparin action in experimental melanoma lung metastasis. *Cancer Res.*, 2004 64(8): 2743-50.

[106] Borsig, L; Wong, R; Feramisco, J; Nadeau, DR; Varki, NM; Varki, A. Heparin and cancer revisited: mechanistic connections involving platelets, P-selectin, carcinoma mucins, and tumor metastasis. *Proc. Natl. Acad. Sci. USA*, 2001 98(6): 3352-7.

[107] Laubli, H; Stevenson, JL; Varki, A; Varki, NM; Borsig, L. L-selectin facilitation of metastasis involves temporal induction of Fut7-dependent ligands at sites of tumor cell arrest. *Cancer Res.*, 2006 66(3): 1536-42.

[108] Borsig, L; Wong, R; Hynes, RO; Varki, NM; Varki, A. Synergistic effects of L- and P-selectin in facilitating tumor metastasis can involve non-mucin ligands and implicate leukocytes as enhancers of metastasis. *Proc. Natl. Acad. Sci. USA*, 2002 99(4): 2193-8.

[109] Fuster, MM; Brown, JR; Wang, L; Esko, JD. A disaccharide precursor of sialyl Lewis X inhibits metastatic potential of tumor cells. *Cancer Res.*, 2003 63(11): 2775-81.

[110] Brown, JR; Fuster, MM; Li, R; Varki, N; Glass, CA; Esko, JD. A disaccharide-based inhibitor of glycosylation attenuates metastatic tumor cell dissemination. *Clin. Cancer Res.*, 2006 12(9): 2894-901.

[111] Brown, JR; Yang, F; Sinha, A; Ramakrishnan, B; Tor, Y; Qasba, PK; Esko, JD. Deoxygenated disaccharide analogs as specific inhibitors of beta1-4-galactosyltransferase 1 and selectin-mediated tumor metastasis. *J. Biol. Chem.*, 2009 284(8): 4952-9.

[112] Fukuda, MN; Ohyama, C; Lowitz, K; Matsuo, O; Pasqualini, R; Ruoslahti, E; Fukuda, M. A peptide mimic of E-selectin ligand inhibits sialyl Lewis X-dependent lung colonization of tumor cells. *Cancer Res.*, 2000 60(2): 450-6.

[113] Nelson, RM; Cecconi, O; Roberts, WG; Aruffo, A; Linhardt, RJ; Bevilacqua, MP. Heparin oligosaccharides bind L- and P-selectin and inhibit acute inflammation. *Blood,* 1993 82(11): 3253-8.

[114] Koenig, A; Norgard-Sumnicht, K; Linhardt, R; Varki, A. Differential interactions of heparin and heparan sulfate glycosaminoglycans with the selectins. Implications for the use of unfractionated and low molecular weight heparins as therapeutic agents. *J. Clin. Invest.*, 1998 101(4): 877-89.

[115] Pineo, GF; Hull, RD. Unfractionated and low-molecular-weight heparin. Comparisons and current recommendations. *Med. Clin. North Am.*, 1998 82(3): 587-99.

[116] Ludwig, RJ; Alban, S; Bistrian, R; Boehncke, WH; Kaufmann, R; Henschler, R; Gille, J. The ability of different forms of heparins to suppress P-selectin function in vitro correlates to their inhibitory capacity on bloodborne metastasis in vivo. *Thromb. Haemost.*, 2006 95(3): 535-40.

[117] Linhardt, RJ; Gunay, NS. Production and chemical processing of low molecular weight heparins. *Semin. Thromb. Hemost.*, 1999 25 Suppl 3: 5-16.

[118] Stevenson, JL; Choi, SH; Varki, A. Differential metastasis inhibition by clinically relevant levels of heparins--correlation with selectin inhibition, not antithrombotic activity. *Clin. Cancer Res.*, 2005 11(19 Pt 1): 7003-11.

[119] Hostettler, N; Naggi, A; Torri, G; Ishai-Michaeli, R; Casu, B; Vlodavsky, I; Borsig, L. P-selectin- and heparanase-dependent

antimetastatic activity of non-anticoagulant heparins. *FASEB J.,* 2007 21(13): 3562-72.

[120] Kragh, M; Binderup, L; Vig Hjarnaa, PJ; Bramm, E; Johansen, KB; Frimundt Petersen, C. Non-anti-coagulant heparin inhibits metastasis but not primary tumor growth. *Oncol. Rep.*, 2005 14(1): 99-104.

[121] Yoshitomi, Y; Nakanishi, H; Kusano, Y; Munesue, S; Oguri, K; Tatematsu, M; Yamashina, I; Okayama, M. Inhibition of experimental lung metastases of Lewis lung carcinoma cells by chemically modified heparin with reduced anticoagulant activity. *Cancer Lett.*, 2004 207(2): 165-74.

[122] Ono, K; Ishihara, M; Ishikawa, K; Ozeki, Y; Deguchi, H; Sato, M; Hashimoto, H; Saito, Y; Yura, H; Kurita, A; Maehara, T. Periodate-treated, non-anticoagulant heparin-carrying polystyrene (NAC-HCPS) affects angiogenesis and inhibits subcutaneous induced tumour growth and metastasis to the lung. *Br. J. Cancer*, 2002 86(11): 1803-12.

[123] Lee, Y; Nam, JH; Shin, HC; Byun, Y. Conjugation of low-molecular-weight heparin and deoxycholic acid for the development of a new oral anticoagulant agent. *Circulation*, 2001 104(25): 3116-20.

[124] Lee, DY; Park, K; Kim, SK; Park, RW; Kwon, IC; Kim, SY; Byun, Y. Antimetastatic effect of an orally active heparin derivative on experimentally induced metastasis. *Clin. Cancer Res.*, 2008 14(9): 2841-9.

[125] Elices, MJ; Osborn, L; Takada, Y; Crouse, C; Luhowskyj, S; Hemler, ME; Lobb, RR. VCAM-1 on activated endothelium interacts with the leukocyte integrin VLA-4 at a site distinct from the VLA-4/fibronectin binding site. *Cell,* 1990 60(4): 577-84.

[126] Klemke, M; Weschenfelder, T; Konstandin, MH; Samstag, Y. High affinity interaction of integrin alpha4beta1 (VLA-4) and vascular cell adhesion molecule 1 (VCAM-1) enhances migration of human melanoma cells across activated endothelial cell layers. *J. Cell Physiol.*, 2007 212(2): 368-74.

[127] Vidal-Vanaclocha, F; Fantuzzi, G; Mendoza, L; Fuentes, AM; Anasagasti, MJ; Martin, J; Carrascal, T; Walsh, P; Reznikov, LL; Kim, SH; Novick, D; Rubinstein, M; Dinarello, CA. IL-18 regulates IL-1beta-dependent hepatic melanoma metastasis via vascular cell adhesion molecule-1. *Proc. Natl. Acad. Sci. USA*, 2000 97(2): 734-9.

[128] Mendoza, L; Carrascal, T; De Luca, M; Fuentes, AM; Salado, C; Blanco, J; Vidal-Vanaclocha, F. Hydrogen peroxide mediates vascular cell adhesion molecule-1 expression from interleukin-18-activated

hepatic sinusoidal endothelium: implications for circulating cancer cell arrest in the murine liver. *Hepatology,* 2001 34(2): 298-310.

[129] Langley, RR; Carlisle, R; Ma, L; Specian, RD; Gerritsen, ME; Granger, DN. Endothelial expression of vascular cell adhesion molecule-1 correlates with metastatic pattern in spontaneous melanoma. *Microcirculation*, 2001 8(5): 335-45.

[130] Schadendorf, D; Heidel, J; Gawlik, C; Suter, L; Czarnetzki, BM. Association with clinical outcome of expression of VLA-4 in primary cutaneous malignant melanoma as well as P-selectin and E-selectin on intratumoral vessels. *J. Natl. Cancer Inst.*, 1995 87(5): 366-71.

[131] Bevilacqua, MP; Nelson, RM. Endothelial-leukocyte adhesion molecules in inflammation and metastasis. *Thromb. Haemost*, 1993 70(1): 152-4.

[132] Natali, P; Nicotra, MR; Cavaliere, R; Bigotti, A; Romano, G; Temponi, M; Ferrone, S. Differential expression of intercellular adhesion molecule 1 in primary and metastatic melanoma lesions. *Cancer Res.*, 1990 50(4): 1271-8.

[133] Haycock, JW; Wagner, M; Morandini, R; Ghanem, G; Rennie, IG; Mac Neil, S. Alpha-melanocyte-stimulating hormone inhibits NF-kappaB activation in human melanocytes and melanoma cells. *J. Invest. Dermatol.*, 1999 113(4): 560-6.

[134] Hedley, SJ; Gawkrodger, DJ; Weetman, AP; Morandini, R; Boeynaems, JM; Ghanem, G; Neil, SM. alpha-Melanocyte stimulating hormone inhibits tumour necrosis factor-alpha stimulated intercellular adhesion molecule-1 expression in normal cutaneous human melanocytes and in melanoma cell lines. *Br. J. Dermatol.*, 1998 138(3): 536-43.

[135] Morandini, R; Boeynaems, JM; Hedley, SJ; MacNeil, S; Ghanem, G. Modulation of ICAM-1 expression by alpha-MSH in human melanoma cells and melanocytes. *J. Cell Physiol.*, 1998 175(3): 276-82.

[136] Zhu, N; Eves, PC; Katerinaki, E; Szabo, M; Morandini, R; Ghanem, G; Lorigan, P; MacNeil, S; Haycock, JW. Melanoma cell attachment, invasion, and integrin expression is upregulated by tumor necrosis factor alpha and suppressed by alpha melanocyte stimulating hormone. *J. Invest. Dermatol.*, 2002 119(5): 1165-71.

[137] Zhu, N; Lalla, R; Eves, P; Brown, TL; King, A; Kemp, EH; Haycock, JW; MacNeil, S. Melanoma cell migration is upregulated by tumour necrosis factor-alpha and suppressed by alpha-melanocyte-stimulating hormone. *Br. J. Cancer*, 2004 90(7): 1457-63.

[138] Katerinaki, E; Evans, GS; Lorigan, PC; MacNeil, S. TNF-alpha increases human melanoma cell invasion and migration in vitro: the role of proteolytic enzymes. *Br. J. Cancer*, 2003 89(6): 1123-9.
[139] Danen, EH; Marcinkiewicz, C; Cornelissen, IM; van Kraats, AA; Pachter, JA; Ruiter, DJ; Niewiarowski, S; van Muijen, GN. The disintegrin eristostatin interferes with integrin alpha 4 beta 1 function and with experimental metastasis of human melanoma cells. *Exp. Cell Res.*, 1998 238(1): 188-96.
[140] Gerritsen, ME; Carley, WW; Ranges, GE; Shen, CP; Phan, SA; Ligon, GF; Perry, CA. Flavonoids inhibit cytokine-induced endothelial cell adhesion protein gene expression. *Am. J. Pathol.*, 1995 147(2): 278-92.
[141] Panes, J; Gerritsen, ME; Anderson, DC; Miyasaka, M; Granger, DN. Apigenin inhibits tumor necrosis factor-induced intercellular adhesion molecule-1 upregulation in vivo. *Microcirculation*, 1996 3(3): 279-86.
[142] Caltagirone, S; Rossi, C; Poggi, A; Ranelletti, FO; Natali, PG; Brunetti, M; Aiello, FB; Piantelli, M. Flavonoids apigenin and quercetin inhibit melanoma growth and metastatic potential. *Int. J. Cancer*, 2000 87(4): 595-600.
[143] Kobuchi, H; Roy, S; Sen, CK; Nguyen, HG; Packer, L. Quercetin inhibits inducible ICAM-1 expression in human endothelial cells through the JNK pathway. *Am. J. Physiol,* 1999 277(3 Pt 1): C403-11.
[144] Ferrer, P; Asensi, M; Segarra, R; Ortega, A; Benlloch, M; Obrador, E; Varea, MT; Asensio, G; Jorda, L; Estrela, JM. Association between pterostilbene and quercetin inhibits metastatic activity of B16 melanoma. *Neoplasia,* 2005 7(1): 37-47.
[145] Guruvayoorappan, C; Kuttan, G. Effect of amentoflavone on the inhibition of pulmonary metastasis induced by B16F-10 melanoma cells in C57BL/6 mice. *Integr. Cancer Ther.*, 2007 6(2): 185-97.
[146] Ramelet, AA. Pharmacologic aspects of a phlebotropic drug in CVI-associated edema. *Angiology*, 2000 51(1): 19-23.
[147] Anderson, PB. Nebulised salbutamol in life-threatening asthma. *Br. Med. J.,* 1979 1(6173): 1284-5.
[148] Nardone, PA; Slotman, GJ; Vezeridis, MP. Ketoconazole: a thromboxane synthetase and 5-lipoxygenase inhibitor with antimetastatic activity in B16-F10 melanoma. *J. Surg. Res.*, 1988 44(4): 425-9.
[149] Lehmann, JM; Holzmann, B; Breitbart, EW; Schmiegelow, P; Riethmuller, G; Johnson, JP. Discrimination between benign and malignant cells of melanocytic lineage by two novel antigens, a

glycoprotein with a molecular weight of 113,000 and a protein with a molecular weight of 76,000. *Cancer Res.,* 1987 47(3): 841-5.

[150] Luca, M; Hunt, B; Bucana, CD; Johnson, JP; Fidler, IJ; Bar-Eli, M. Direct correlation between MUC18 expression and metastatic potential of human melanoma cells. *Melanoma Res.*, 1993 3(1): 35-41.

[151] Xie, S; Luca, M; Huang, S; Gutman, M; Reich, R; Johnson, JP; Bar-Eli, M. Expression of MCAM/MUC18 by human melanoma cells leads to increased tumor growth and metastasis. *Cancer Res.*, 1997 57(11): 2295-303.

[152] Mills, L; Tellez, C; Huang, S; Baker, C; McCarty, M; Green, L; Gudas, JM; Feng, X; Bar-Eli, M. Fully human antibodies to MCAM/MUC18 inhibit tumor growth and metastasis of human melanoma. *Cancer Res.*, 2002 62(17): 5106-14.

[153] Psaila, B; Kaplan, RN; Port, ER; Lyden, D. Priming the 'soil' for breast cancer metastasis: the pre-metastatic niche. *Breast Dis.*, 2006 26: 65-74.

[154] Braun, S; Vogl, FD; Naume, B; Janni, W; Osborne, MP; Coombes, RC; Schlimok, G; Diel, IJ; Gerber, B; Gebauer, G; Pierga, JY; Marth, C; Oruzio, D; Wiedswang, G; Solomayer, EF; Kundt, G; Strobl, B; Fehm, T; Wong, GY; Bliss, J; Vincent-Salomon, A; Pantel, K. A pooled analysis of bone marrow micrometastasis in breast cancer. *N. Engl. J. Med.*, 2005 353(8): 793-802.

[155] Dittmar, T; Heyder, C; Gloria-Maercker, E; Hatzmann, W; Zanker, KS. Adhesion molecules and chemokines: the navigation system for circulating tumor (stem) cells to metastasize in an organ-specific manner. *Clin. Exp. Metastasis*, 2008 25(1): 11-32.

[156] Richmond, A; Yang, J; Su, Y. The good and the bad of chemokines/chemokine receptors in melanoma. *Pigment Cell Melanoma Res.*, 2009 22(2): 175-86.

[157] Robledo, MM; Bartolome, RA; Longo, N; Rodriguez-Frade, JM; Mellado, M; Longo, I; van Muijen, GN; Sanchez-Mateos, P; Teixido, J. Expression of functional chemokine receptors CXCR3 and CXCR4 on human melanoma cells. *J. Biol. Chem.*, 2001 276(48): 45098-105.

[158] Muller, A; Homey, B; Soto, H; Ge, N; Catron, D; Buchanan, ME; McClanahan, T; Murphy, E; Yuan, W; Wagner, SN; Barrera, JL; Mohar, A; Verastegui, E; Zlotnik, A. Involvement of chemokine receptors in breast cancer metastasis. *Nature,* 2001 410(6824): 50-6.

[159] Geminder, H; Sagi-Assif, O; Goldberg, L; Meshel, T; Rechavi, G; Witz, IP; Ben-Baruch, A. A possible role for CXCR4 and its ligand, the CXC chemokine stromal cell-derived factor-1, in the development of bone

marrow metastases in neuroblastoma. *J. Immunol.*, 2001 167(8): 4747-57.

[160] Murakami, T; Maki, W; Cardones, AR; Fang, H; Tun Kyi, A; Nestle, FO; Hwang, ST. Expression of CXC chemokine receptor-4 enhances the pulmonary metastatic potential of murine B16 melanoma cells. *Cancer Res.*, 2002 62(24): 7328-34.

[161] Scala, S; Giuliano, P; Ascierto, PA; Ierano, C; Franco, R; Napolitano, M; Ottaiano, A; Lombardi, ML; Luongo, M; Simeone, E; Castiglia, D; Mauro, F; De Michele, I; Calemma, R; Botti, G; Caraco, C; Nicoletti, G; Satriano, RA; Castello, G. Human melanoma metastases express functional CXCR4. *Clin. Cancer Res.*, 2006 12(8): 2427-33.

[162] Kim, J; Mori, T; Chen, SL; Amersi, FF; Martinez, SR; Kuo, C; Turner, RR; Ye, X; Bilchik, AJ; Morton, DL; Hoon, DS. Chemokine receptor CXCR4 expression in patients with melanoma and colorectal cancer liver metastases and the association with disease outcome. *Ann. Surg.*, 2006 244(1): 113-20.

[163] Cardones, AR; Murakami, T; Hwang, ST. CXCR4 enhances adhesion of B16 tumor cells to endothelial cells in vitro and in vivo via beta(1) integrin. *Cancer Res.*, 2003 63(20): 6751-7.

[164] Scala, S; Ottaiano, A; Ascierto, PA; Cavalli, M; Simeone, E; Giuliano, P; Napolitano, M; Franco, R; Botti, G; Castello, G. Expression of CXCR4 predicts poor prognosis in patients with malignant melanoma. *Clin. Cancer Res.*, 2005 11(5): 1835-41.

[165] Bartolome, RA; Ferreiro, S; Miquilena-Colina, ME; Martinez-Prats, L; Soto-Montenegro, ML; Garcia-Bernal, D; Vaquero, JJ; Agami, R; Delgado, R; Desco, M; Sanchez-Mateos, P; Teixido, J. The chemokine receptor CXCR4 and the metalloproteinase MT1-MMP are mutually required during melanoma metastasis to lungs. *Am. J. Pathol.*, 2009 174(2): 602-12.

[166] Murphy, PM. Chemokines and the molecular basis of cancer metastasis. *N. Engl. J. Med.,* 2001 345(11): 833-5.

[167] Yan, L; Anderson, GM; DeWitte, M; Nakada, MT. Therapeutic potential of cytokine and chemokine antagonists in cancer therapy. *Eur. J. Cancer*, 2006 42(6): 793-802.

[168] Nakashima, H; Masuda, M; Murakami, T; Koyanagi, Y; Matsumoto, A; Fujii, N; Yamamoto, N. Anti-human immunodeficiency virus activity of a novel synthetic peptide, T22 ([Tyr-5,12, Lys-7]polyphemusin II): a possible inhibitor of virus-cell fusion. *Antimicrob. Agents Chemother.*, 1992 36(6): 1249-55.

[169] Tamamura, H; Xu, Y; Hattori, T; Zhang, X; Arakaki, R; Kanbara, K; Omagari, A; Otaka, A; Ibuka, T; Yamamoto, N; Nakashima, H; Fujii, N. A low-molecular-weight inhibitor against the chemokine receptor CXCR4: a strong anti-HIV peptide T140. *Biochem. Biophys. Res. Commun.*, 1998 253(3): 877-82.

[170] Tamamura, H; Hori, A; Kanzaki, N; Hiramatsu, K; Mizumoto, M; Nakashima, H; Yamamoto, N; Otaka, A; Fujii, N. T140 analogs as CXCR4 antagonists identified as anti-metastatic agents in the treatment of breast cancer. *FEBS Lett.*, 2003 550(1-3): 79-83.

[171] Tamamura, H; Omagari, A; Hiramatsu, K; Gotoh, K; Kanamoto, T; Xu, Y; Kodama, E; Matsuoka, M; Hattori, T; Yamamoto, N; Nakashima, H; Otaka, A; Fujii, N. Development of specific CXCR4 inhibitors possessing high selectivity indexes as well as complete stability in serum based on an anti-HIV peptide T140. *Bioorg. Med. Chem. Lett.,* 2001 11(14): 1897-902.

[172] Mori, T; Doi, R; Koizumi, M; Toyoda, E; Ito, D; Kami, K; Masui, T; Fujimoto, K; Tamamura, H; Hiramatsu, K; Fujii, N; Imamura, M. CXCR4 antagonist inhibits stromal cell-derived factor 1-induced migration and invasion of human pancreatic cancer. *Mol. Cancer Ther.*, 2004 3(1): 29-37.

[173] Liang, Z; Wu, T; Lou, H; Yu, X; Taichman, RS; Lau, SK; Nie, S; Umbreit, J; Shim, H. Inhibition of breast cancer metastasis by selective synthetic polypeptide against CXCR4. *Cancer Res.*, 2004 64(12): 4302-8.

[174] Takenaga, M; Tamamura, H; Hiramatsu, K; Nakamura, N; Yamaguchi, Y; Kitagawa, A; Kawai, S; Nakashima, H; Fujii, N; Igarashi, R. A single treatment with microcapsules containing a CXCR4 antagonist suppresses pulmonary metastasis of murine melanoma. *Biochem. Biophys. Res. Commun.*, 2004 320(1): 226-32.

[175] Kim, SY; Lee, CH; Midura, BV; Yeung, C; Mendoza, A; Hong, SH; Ren, L; Wong, D; Korz, W; Merzouk, A; Salari, H; Zhang, H; Hwang, ST; Khanna, C; Helman, LJ. Inhibition of the CXCR4/CXCL12 chemokine pathway reduces the development of murine pulmonary metastases. *Clin. Exp. Metastasis*, 2008 25(3): 201-11.

[176] Bridger, GJ; Skerlj, RT; Thornton, D; Padmanabhan, S; Martellucci, SA; Henson, GW; Abrams, MJ; Yamamoto, N; De Vreese, K; Pauwels, R; et al. Synthesis and structure-activity relationships of phenylenebis(methylene)-linked bis-tetraazamacrocycles that inhibit

HIV replication. Effects of macrocyclic ring size and substituents on the aromatic linker. *J. Med. Chem.*, 1995 38(2): 366-78.

[177] De Clercq, E. Potential clinical applications of the CXCR4 antagonist bicyclam AMD3100. *Mini. Rev. Med. Chem.*, 2005 5(9): 805-24.

[178] Li, JK; Yu, L; Shen, Y; Zhou, LS; Wang, YC; Zhang, JH. Inhibition of CXCR4 activity with AMD3100 decreases invasion of human colorectal cancer cells in vitro. *World J. Gastroenterol.,* 2008 14(15): 2308-13.

[179] Matsusue, R; Kubo, H; Hisamori, S; Okoshi, K; Takagi, H; Hida, K; Nakano, K; Itami, A; Kawada, K; Nagayama, S; Sakai, Y. Hepatic stellate cells promote liver metastasis of colon cancer cells by the action of SDF-1/CXCR4 axis. *Ann. Surg. Oncol.*, 2009 16(9): 2645-53.

[180] De Clercq, E. The bicyclam AMD3100 story. *Nat. Rev. Drug Discov.*, 2003 2(7): 581-7.

[181] Kawada, K; Sonoshita, M; Sakashita, H; Takabayashi, A; Yamaoka, Y; Manabe, T; Inaba, K; Minato, N; Oshima, M; Taketo, MM. Pivotal role of CXCR3 in melanoma cell metastasis to lymph nodes. *Cancer Res.,* 2004 64(11): 4010-7.

[182] Monteagudo, C; Martin, JM; Jorda, E; Llombart-Bosch, A. CXCR3 chemokine receptor immunoreactivity in primary cutaneous malignant melanoma: correlation with clinicopathological prognostic factors. *J. Clin. Pathol.*, 2007 60(6): 596-9.

[183] Walser, TC; Rifat, S; Ma, X; Kundu, N; Ward, C; Goloubeva, O; Johnson, MG; Medina, JC; Collins, TL; Fulton, AM. Antagonism of CXCR3 inhibits lung metastasis in a murine model of metastatic breast cancer. *Cancer Res.*, 2006 66(15): 7701-7.

[184] Cambien, B; Karimdjee, BF; Richard-Fiardo, P; Bziouech, H; Barthel, R; Millet, MA; Martini, V; Birnbaum, D; Scoazec, JY; Abello, J; Al Saati, T; Johnson, MG; Sullivan, TJ; Medina, JC; Collins, TL; Schmid-Alliana, A; Schmid-Antomarchi, H. Organ-specific inhibition of metastatic colon carcinoma by CXCR3 antagonism. *Br. J. Cancer,* 2009 100(11): 1755-64.

[185] Pradelli, E; Karimdjee-Soilihi, B; Michiels, JF; Ricci, JE; Millet, MA; Vandenbos, F; Sullivan, TJ; Collins, TL; Johnson, MG; Medina, JC; Kleinerman, ES; Schmid-Alliana, A; Schmid-Antomarchi, H. Antagonism of chemokine receptor CXCR3 inhibits osteosarcoma metastasis to lungs. *Int. J. Cancer*, 2009 125(11): 2586-94.

[186] Amersi, FF; Terando, AM; Goto, Y; Scolyer, RA; Thompson, JF; Tran, AN; Faries, MB; Morton, DL; Hoon, DS. Activation of CCR9/CCL25 in

cutaneous melanoma mediates preferential metastasis to the small intestine. *Clin. Cancer Res.*, 2008 14(3): 638-45.

[187] Eksteen, B; Adams, DH. GSK-1605786, a selective small-molecule antagonist of the CCR9 chemokine receptor for the treatment of Crohn's disease. *IDrugs,* 2010 13(7): 472-781.

[188] Kaplan, RN; Riba, RD; Zacharoulis, S; Bramley, AH; Vincent, L; Costa, C; MacDonald, DD; Jin, DK; Shido, K; Kerns, SA; Zhu, Z; Hicklin, D; Wu, Y; Port, JL; Altorki, N; Port, ER; Ruggero, D; Shmelkov, SV; Jensen, KK; Rafii, S; Lyden, D. VEGFR1-positive haematopoietic bone marrow progenitors initiate the pre-metastatic niche. *Nature,* 2005 438(7069): 820-7.

[189] Kaplan, RN; Psaila, B; Lyden, D. Bone marrow cells in the 'pre-metastatic niche': within bone and beyond. *Cancer Metastasis Rev.*, 2006 25(4): 521-9.

[190] Kaplan, RN; Rafii, S; Lyden, D. Preparing the "soil": the premetastatic niche. *Cancer Res.*, 2006 66(23): 11089-93.

[191] Li, L; Neaves, WB. Normal stem cells and cancer stem cells: the niche matters. *Cancer Res.*, 2006 66(9): 4553-7.

[192] Naumov, GN; Akslen, LA; Folkman, J. Role of angiogenesis in human tumor dormancy: animal models of the angiogenic switch. *Cell Cycle*, 2006 5(16): 1779-87.

[193] Li, HC; Stoicov, C; Rogers, AB; Houghton, J. Stem cells and cancer: evidence for bone marrow stem cells in epithelial cancers. *World J. Gastroenterol.*, 2006 12(3): 363-71.

[194] Perret, GY. Pharmacological strategies and micrometastasis: what is known? What must be done? *Minerva Med.*, 2010 101(3): 163-78.

[195] Wiley, HE; Gonzalez, EB; Maki, W; Wu, MT; Hwang, ST. Expression of CC chemokine receptor-7 and regional lymph node metastasis of B16 murine melanoma. *J. Natl. Cancer Inst.*, 2001 93(21): 1638-43.

[196] Takeuchi, H; Fujimoto, A; Tanaka, M; Yamano, T; Hsueh, E; Hoon, DS. CCL21 chemokine regulates chemokine receptor CCR7 bearing malignant melanoma cells. *Clin. Cancer Res.*, 2004 10(7): 2351-8.

[197] Lanati, S; Dunn, DB; Roussigne, M; Emmett, MS; Carriere, V; Jullien, D; Budge, J; Fryer, J; Erard, M; Cailler, F; Girard, JP; Bates, DO. Chemotrap-1: An Engineered Soluble Receptor That Blocks Chemokine-Induced Migration of Metastatic Cancer Cells In vivo. *Cancer Res.,* 2010 70(20): 8138-48.

[198] Vermeulen, PB; van Golen, KL; Dirix, LY. Angiogenesis, lymphangiogenesis, growth pattern, and tumor emboli in inflammatory

breast cancer: a review of the current knowledge. *Cancer,* 2010 116(11 Suppl): 2748-54.

[199] Zetter, BR. Angiogenesis and tumor metastasis. *Annu. Rev. Med.*, 1998 49: 407-24.

[200] Borges, E; Jan, Y; Ruoslahti, E. Platelet-derived growth factor receptor beta and vascular endothelial growth factor receptor 2 bind to the beta 3 integrin through its extracellular domain. *J. Biol. Chem.*, 2000 275(51): 39867-73.

[201] Soldi, R; Mitola, S; Strasly, M; Defilippi, P; Tarone, G; Bussolino, F. Role of alphavbeta3 integrin in the activation of vascular endothelial growth factor receptor-2. *EMBO J.,* 1999 18(4): 882-92.

[202] Garanger, E; Boturyn, D; Dumy, P. Tumor targeting with RGD peptide ligands-design of new molecular conjugates for imaging and therapy of cancers. *Anticancer Agents Med. Chem.*, 2007 7(5): 552-8.

[203] Brooks, PC; Clark, RA; Cheresh, DA. Requirement of vascular integrin alpha v beta 3 for angiogenesis. *Science,* 1994 264(5158): 569-71.

[204] Frelinger, AL, 3rd; Cohen, I; Plow, EF; Smith, MA; Roberts, J; Lam, SC; Ginsberg, MH. Selective inhibition of integrin function by antibodies specific for ligand-occupied receptor conformers. *J. Biol. Chem.*, 1990 265(11): 6346-52.

[205] Smith, JW; Vestal, DJ; Irwin, SV; Burke, TA; Cheresh, DA. Purification and functional characterization of integrin alpha v beta 5. An adhesion receptor for vitronectin. *J. Biol. Chem.*, 1990 265(19): 11008-13.

[206] Coleman, KR; Braden, GA; Willingham, MC; Sane, DC. Vitaxin, a humanized monoclonal antibody to the vitronectin receptor (alphavbeta3), reduces neointimal hyperplasia and total vessel area after balloon injury in hypercholesterolemic rabbits. *Circ. Res.*, 1999 84(11): 1268-76.

[207] Posey, JA; Khazaeli, MB; DelGrosso, A; Saleh, MN; Lin, CY; Huse, W; LoBuglio, AF. A pilot trial of Vitaxin, a humanized anti-vitronectin receptor (anti alpha v beta 3) antibody in patients with metastatic cancer. *Cancer Biother. Radiopharm.*, 2001 16(2): 125-32.

[208] Tucker, GC. Integrins: molecular targets in cancer therapy. *Curr. Oncol. Rep.*, 2006 8(2): 96-103.

[209] Mikecz, K. Vitaxin applied molecular evolution. *Curr. Opin. Investig Drugs*, 2000 1(2): 199-203.

[210] Gutheil, JC; Campbell, TN; Pierce, PR; Watkins, JD; Huse, WD; Bodkin, DJ; Cheresh, DA. Targeted antiangiogenic therapy for cancer

using Vitaxin: a humanized monoclonal antibody to the integrin alphavbeta3. *Clin. Cancer Res.*, 2000 6(8): 3056-61.

[211] Harms, JF; Welch, DR; Samant, RS; Shevde, LA; Miele, ME; Babu, GR; Goldberg, SF; Gilman, VR; Sosnowski, DM; Campo, DA; Gay, CV; Budgeon, LR; Mercer, R; Jewell, J; Mastro, AM; Donahue, HJ; Erin, N; Debies, MT; Meehan, WJ; Jones, AL; Mbalaviele, G; Nickols, A; Christensen, ND; Melly, R; Beck, LN; Kent, J; Rader, RK; Kotyk, JJ; Pagel, MD; Westlin, WF; Griggs, DW. A small molecule antagonist of the alpha(v)beta3 integrin suppresses MDA-MB-435 skeletal metastasis. *Clin. Exp. Metastasis*, 2004 21(2): 119-28.

[212] Maubant, S; Saint-Dizier, D; Boutillon, M; Perron-Sierra, F; Casara, PJ; Hickman, JA; Tucker, GC; Van Obberghen-Schilling, E. Blockade of alpha v beta3 and alpha v beta5 integrins by RGD mimetics induces anoikis and not integrin-mediated death in human endothelial cells. *Blood,* 2006 108(9): 3035-44.

[213] Reinmuth, N; Liu, W; Ahmad, SA; Fan, F; Stoeltzing, O; Parikh, AA; Bucana, CD; Gallick, GE; Nickols, MA; Westlin, WF; Ellis, LM. Alphavbeta3 integrin antagonist S247 decreases colon cancer metastasis and angiogenesis and improves survival in mice. *Cancer Res.*, 2003 63(9): 2079-87.

[214] Shannon, KE; Keene, JL; Settle, SL; Duffin, TD; Nickols, MA; Westlin, M; Schroeter, S; Ruminski, PG; Griggs, DW. Anti-metastatic properties of RGD-peptidomimetic agents S137 and S247. *Clin. Exp. Metastasis*, 2004 21(2): 129-38.

[215] Smith, JW. Cilengitide Merck. *Curr. Opin. Investig. Drugs*, 2003 4(6): 741-5.

[216] Nisato, RE; Tille, JC; Jonczyk, A; Goodman, SL; Pepper, MS. alphav beta 3 and alphav beta 5 integrin antagonists inhibit angiogenesis in vitro. *Angiogenesis*, 2003 6(2): 105-19.

[217] Yamada, S; Bu, XY; Khankaldyyan, V; Gonzales-Gomez, I; McComb, JG; Laug, WE. Effect of the angiogenesis inhibitor Cilengitide (EMD 121974) on glioblastoma growth in nude mice. *Neurosurgery*, 2006 59(6): 1304-12; discussion 1312.

[218] Buerkle, MA; Pahernik, SA; Sutter, A; Jonczyk, A; Messmer, K; Dellian, M. Inhibition of the alpha-nu integrins with a cyclic RGD peptide impairs angiogenesis, growth and metastasis of solid tumours in vivo. *Br. J. Cancer*, 2002 86(5): 788-95.

[219] Bieler, G; Hasmim, M; Monnier, Y; Imaizumi, N; Ameyar, M; Bamat, J; Ponsonnet, L; Chouaib, S; Grell, M; Goodman, SL; Lejeune, F; Ruegg,

C. Distinctive role of integrin-mediated adhesion in TNF-induced PKB/Akt and NF-kappaB activation and endothelial cell survival. *Oncogene*, 2007 26(39): 5722-32.

[220] Tentori, L; Dorio, AS; Muzi, A; Lacal, PM; Ruffini, F; Navarra, P; Graziani, G. The integrin antagonist cilengitide increases the antitumor activity of temozolomide against malignant melanoma. *Oncol. Rep.*, 2008 19(4): 1039-43.

[221] Albert, JM; Cao, C; Geng, L; Leavitt, L; Hallahan, DE; Lu, B. Integrin alpha v beta 3 antagonist Cilengitide enhances efficacy of radiotherapy in endothelial cell and non-small-cell lung cancer models. *Int. J. Radiat. Oncol. Biol. Phys.*, 2006 65(5): 1536-43.

[222] Raguse, JD; Gath, HJ; Bier, J; Riess, H; Oettle, H. Cilengitide (EMD 121974) arrests the growth of a heavily pretreated highly vascularised head and neck tumour. *Oral. Oncol.*, 2004 40(2): 228-30.

[223] Friess, H; Langrehr, JM; Oettle, H; Raedle, J; Niedergethmann, M; Dittrich, C; Hossfeld, DK; Stoger, H; Neyns, B; Herzog, P; Piedbois, P; Dobrowolski, F; Scheithauer, W; Hawkins, R; Katz, F; Balcke, P; Vermorken, J; van Belle, S; Davidson, N; Esteve, AA; Castellano, D; Kleeff, J; Tempia-Caliera, AA; Kovar, A; Nippgen, J. A randomized multi-center phase II trial of the angiogenesis inhibitor Cilengitide (EMD 121974) and gemcitabine compared with gemcitabine alone in advanced unresectable pancreatic cancer. *BMC Cancer*, 2006 6: 285.

[224] Alghisi, GC; Ponsonnet, L; Ruegg, C. The integrin antagonist cilengitide activates alphaVbeta3, disrupts VE-cadherin localization at cell junctions and enhances permeability in endothelial cells. *PLoS One*, 2009 4(2): e4449.

[225] Jiang, C; Agarwal, R; Lu, J. Anti-angiogenic potential of a cancer chemopreventive flavonoid antioxidant, silymarin: inhibition of key attributes of vascular endothelial cells and angiogenic cytokine secretion by cancer epithelial cells. *Biochem. Biophys. Res. Commun.*, 2000 276(1): 371-8.

[226] Zi, X; Feyes, DK; Agarwal, R. Anticarcinogenic effect of a flavonoid antioxidant, silymarin, in human breast cancer cells MDA-MB 468: induction of G1 arrest through an increase in Cip1/p21 concomitant with a decrease in kinase activity of cyclin-dependent kinases and associated cyclins. *Clin. Cancer Res.*, 1998 4(4): 1055-64.

[227] Deep, G; Singh, RP; Agarwal, C; Kroll, DJ; Agarwal, R. Silymarin and silibinin cause G1 and G2-M cell cycle arrest via distinct circuitries in

human prostate cancer PC3 cells: a comparison of flavanone silibinin with flavanolignan mixture silymarin. *Oncogene*, 2006 25(7): 1053-69.
[228] Yang, SH; Lin, JK; Chen, WS; Chiu, JH. Anti-angiogenic effect of silymarin on colon cancer LoVo cell line. *J. Surg. Res.*, 2003 113(1): 133-8.
[229] Lah, JJ; Cui, W; Hu, KQ. Effects and mechanisms of silibinin on human hepatoma cell lines. *World J. Gastroenterol.*, 2007 13(40): 5299-305.
[230] Singh, RP; Deep, G; Chittezhath, M; Kaur, M; Dwyer-Nield, LD; Malkinson, AM; Agarwal, R. Effect of silibinin on the growth and progression of primary lung tumors in mice. *J. Natl. Cancer Inst.*, 2006 98(12): 846-55.
[231] Agarwal, R; Agarwal, C; Ichikawa, H; Singh, RP; Aggarwal, BB. Anticancer potential of silymarin: from bench to bed side. *Anticancer Res.*, 2006 26(6B): 4457-98.
[232] Yamagishi, S; Abe, R; Inagaki, Y; Nakamura, K; Sugawara, H; Inokuma, D; Nakamura, H; Shimizu, T; Takeuchi, M; Yoshimura, A; Bucala, R; Shimizu, H; Imaizumi, T. Minodronate, a newly developed nitrogen-containing bisphosphonate, suppresses melanoma growth and improves survival in nude mice by blocking vascular endothelial growth factor signaling. *Am. J. Pathol.*, 2004 165(6): 1865-74.

In: Metastatic Melanoma
Editors: S.A. Klein and J.P. Beckler
ISBN 978-1-61209-915-6

Chapter II

Invasion and Metastasis: Major Obstacles to Curative Cancer Therapy

Girija Kuttan* and P. Pratheeshkumar
Amala Cancer Research Centre, Amala Nagar,
Thrissur-680555, Kerala State, India

Abstract

Cancer is a major health problem and is the second leading cause of death in the world. Invasion and metastasis are the greatest obstacles to the successful tumour treatment. Metastasis is a multi-stage process involving adhesion of the cancer cells to the basement membrane, invasion through the basement membrane, cancer cell motility, intravasation, transit in the blood or lymph, extravasation and growth at a new site. Any drug, which can inhibit one of the steps in the cascade, will be useful in the inhibition of tumour metastasis. Death from cancer is most often due to metastases that are resistant to conventional therapies. Although there are several drugs available to encounter cancer growth in humans, there are no drugs presently available to specifically inhibit the

* Ph. No. 91-487-2307968, Fax: 91-487-2307968, E-mail : girijakuttan@gmail.com.

metastasis of cancer cells. This review focuses on metastatic cascade and possible therapeutic targets.

Keywords: Metastatic cascade; Angiogenesis; Matrix Metalloproteases; Vascular endothelial growth factor; Metastasis suppressor genes; Hypoxia and metastasis; NF-κB and metastasis; Nitric oxide and metastasis; Apoptosis and metastasis; Current therapies; Therapeutic targets.

Introduction

Cancer is a hyperproliferative disorder recognised to be a second major health problem in the world. Tumour metastasis is the leading cause of cancer-related morbidity and mortality. Invasion and metastasis are hallmarks of tumour malignancy and major obstacles to curative cancer therapies. Metastasis is the process by which a tumour cell leaves the primary tumour, travels to a distant site via the circulatory system, and establishes a secondary tumour. Cancer metastasis consists of multiple, complex, interacting, and interdependent steps, requiring invasion from the primary tumour, intravasation, survival, arrest and extravasation of the circulatory system and colonization of a distant site. Each step in the process is rate-limiting; failure to complete any one prevents the tumour cell from producing a metastasis (Palmieri et al., 2007, Ellis and Fidler, 1996), but the majority of the tumour cells fail to survive and establish a metastatic cascade, which is termed metastatic inefficiency.

Tumour Cell Metastasis - Metastatic Cascade

To successfully colonize a distant organ, a tumour cell must complete all steps of the cascade. Failure to complete any step results in the failure to colonize metastatic target organs. Major steps involved in the cascade are as follows:

a) Detachment of cells from primary tumour
b) Tumour cell invasion
c) Intravasation
d) Cancer cells in the blood stream
e) Extravasation
f) Implantation into target organ
g) Tumour angiogenesis

Detachment of Cells from Primary Tumour

Detachment of cells of the primary tumour and the adhesion of tumour cells on a distant site are considered to be the crucial steps in the metastasis cascade. Tumour cells often show a decrease in cell-cell and/or cell-matrix adhesion. An increasing body of evidence indicates that this reduction in cell adhesion correlates with tumour invasion and metastasis (Cavallaro and Christofori, 2001). Tumour cells isolated from metastases are highly migratory and invasive. Evidence suggests that the surfaces of tumour cells may differ from those of homologous normal cells. Cancer cells carry rich content of N-acetyl neuraminic acid (Neu5Ac or NANA) on the surface, showing high negative charge that reduces cell-cell adhesion. Metastatic cancer cells often express a high density of sialic acid-rich glycoproteins. Experiments proved that supplement of L-glutamine enhance the synthesis of a key intermediate in the formation of the cell surface carbohydrates required for adhesion (Oppenheimer et al., 1969). Cancer cells secrete some powerful proteolytic enzymes (protease) that also reduce cell-cell adhesion which leads to the cell detachment from primary tumour, evidence that protease inhibitors can block the cancer cell detachments (Meyer et al., 1983). Some tumour cells exist as cell suspensions, they do not adhere at all. These cells do not have the cell surface carbohydrates required for cell adhesion.

The shape of cells is determined by the cytoskeleton. Defects in the cytoskeleton in some cancer cells may cause them to round up and break adhesive bonds. Defective cytoskeleton, altered surface carbohydrates and excessive protease production appear to weaken adhesive bonds in primary tumours in preparation for cancer spread (Cavallaro and Christofori, 2001). Tumour tissue is deficient in calcium which has for long been considered to be important in the establishment of inter-cellular adhesions. Experiments showed that the cancer cells usually contained about half the amount of calcium than did the normal cells from the same tissue, low calcium concentration is an important factor in the weaker adhesion of cancer cells (Coman, 1944, Coman, 1953).

Adhesion Molecules and Receptors

Cell adhesion is a vital process, essential for the establishment and maintenance of tissue architecture and differentiation. Adhesion between adjacent cells or between cells and the surrounding extracellular matrix is critical in the dynamic processes necessary for tissue morphogenesis in embryos and in the maintenance of complex differentiated tissues in adult organisms (Ramburan and Govender, 2002). Cell adhesion molecules (CAMs) are cell surface glycoprotein that mediates the physical interactions between adjacent cells and between cells and the surrounding extracellular matrix. CAMs belong to different protein families, depending on their structural and functional properties (Francavilla et al., 2009). They are involved in the regulation of both physiological and pathophysiological processes, such as development, growth, tissue homeostasis, immune responses, wound healing, inflammation and neoplasia. Their fundamental role is to maintain tissue integrity and to regulate cell movement and migration in both a temporal and spatial sense (Thomas et al., 1997). Malignant tumours are characterised by unrestrained cellular growth, invasion of adjacent tissue and their ability to metastasise. Alterations in cell surface receptors and adhesion molecules which regulate cell-cell and cell-matrix interactions have been implicated in these tumour processes (Albelda, 1993). There are four major groups of cell adhesion molecules (CAMs); cadherins, integrins, immunoglobulin superfamily, and selectins. Table 1 show important cell adhesion molecules and their ligands (Castells and Rustgi, 2003).

Cadherins

Cadherins are a large family of cell adhesion molecules, which mediate cell-cell adhesion via calcium dependent, homotypic interactions. These molecules have intra- and extracellular domains, which are integral to the mechanism of cell adhesion. The intracellular domains interact with catenins, which link the cadherins to the actin cytoskeleton. Alterations in either of these groups of molecules have been identified as key mechanisms in various disease processes. Complex alterations in adhesion have been proposed as a requirement for tumour invasion and metastases (Ramburan and Govender, 2002). The cadherins are sub divided into classical and desmosomal subtypes.

Table 1. Cell adhesion molecules and their ligands

Cadherins		**IgG superfamily**	
N-cadherin	Homophilic binding	ICAM-1	$\alpha_L\ \beta_2$
E-cadherin	Homophilic binding	ICAM-2	$\alpha_L\ \beta_2$
P-cadherin	Homophilic binding	ICAM-3	$\alpha_L\ \beta_2$
Integrins		VCAM-1	$\alpha_4\ \beta_2$
$\alpha_1\beta_1$	Collagens, laminin	LFA-2	LFA-3
$\alpha_2\ \beta_1$	Collagens, laminin,	LFA-3	LFA-2
fibronectin		N-CAM	Neural and glial
$\alpha_3\ \beta_1$	Collagen 1,	cells	
fibronectin		**Selectins**	
$\alpha_4\ \beta_1$	Fibronectin, VCAM	E-selectin	Sialyl–Lewis X
$\alpha_5\ \beta_1$	Fibronectin	L-selectin	Carbohydrate
$\alpha_6\ \beta_1$	Laminin	P-selectin	Lewis X (CD15)
$\alpha_L\ \beta_2$	Fibrinogen, ICAM	**Others**	
$\alpha_M\ \beta_2$	Fibrinogen, ICAM,	CD44 and isoforms	Hyaluronic acid,
factor X			laminin,
$\alpha_X\ \beta_2$	Fibrinogen, C3bi	collagens	
		67-kDa laminin receptor	Laminin

Classical cadherins are characterized by a highly conserved cytoplasmic domain and the ability to form complexes through very specifc interactions with intracellular proteins called catenins. Catenins, in turn, link cadherins to the actin filament network. These catenins, along with the cadherin molecule, localize to the zonula adherens of the cell and participate in junction formation and stabilization. The classical cadherins include E (epithelial)-, N (neuronal)-, P (placental)-, and VE (vascular endothelial)- cadherin (Ramburan and Govender, 2002).

E-cadherin is the key component for adherence junctions between epithelial cells, and one of the best characterised cadherins. Induction of Ca^{2+}-dependent cell–cell contact results in the rapid localization of surface E-cadherin molecules to the regions of contact where it extracellularly forms homophilic junctions with neighboring cells (Shiozaki et al., 1996, Bremnes et al., 2002). E-cadherin was identified as a metastasis suppressor molecule in carcinomas. This has been confirmed by numerous descriptive and experimental studies and is now a well-accepted paradigm (Starzinski-Powitz et al., 1999). Over-expression of E-cadherin in cancer cells decrease motility and invasion. Also, loss of E-cadherin has been associated with increased cancer invasion. The primary proposed mechanism of E-cadherin in cancer metastasis is to inhibit cell shedding from the primary tumor. E-cadherin prevents cellular detachment from the primary tumour mass and intravasation, thereby blocking any entry into the metastatic cascade (Prodromou et al., 1999). E-cadherin is bound to the actin cytoskeleton via a series of proteins, the catenins. Catenins have been classified into α-, β- and γ –catenin. In normal epithelial cells and non metastatic carcinomas, E-cadherin can form two complexes with catenins. One complex comprises E-cadherin, β-catenin and α-catenin, and in the other, β-catenin is replaced by plakoglobin (also called γ -catenin). These interactions are necessary for E-cadherin function (Aberle et al., 1996). Alteration of the functionally active catenins results in loss of the ability of E-cadherin to establish cell-cell adhesion. Moreover loss of function of E-cadherin correlates with increased invasiveness and metastasis of tumours. N-cadherin (neural) is expressed in neural tissue, smooth muscle, fibroblasts and endothelial cells, and has a demonstrated role as a metastasis suppressor, which when over-expressed in the LM8 osteosarcoma line, inhibited pulmonary metastasis (Kashima et al., 2003). However, other data show that N-cadherin increases aggressiveness and metastasis in breast and melanoma cell lines (Stafford et al., 2008). P-cadherin (placental) present in the placenta, lung epithelium, skin and myoepithelial mammary cells, and is highly expressed in epithelial cells with proliferative capability and decreases as cells differentiate. VE cadherin (vascular endothelial) is specifically located in endothelial cells (Paschos et al., 2009). In general, cadherin genes are regarded as tumour suppressors and their deficient expression favours neoplastic progression (Okegawa et al., 2004).

Desmosomal cadherins are the transmembrane protein components of desmosomes. Desmosomes are sites of cell-cell adhesion present in tissues subject to mechanical stress, such as the epidermis and the myocardium. Desmocollin and desmoglein, are the major adhesion molecules of desmosomes. The main difference from classical cadherins is found in the cytoplasmic domain of desmosomal cadherins that interact not with β-catenins but with a different group of cytoplasmic adapter proteins including desmoplakin, plakophillin and plakoglobin. Desmosomes have been shown to have a role in tumour suppression similar to E-cadherin (Tselepis et al., 1998).

Integrins

The integrins are a family of transmembrane linker proteins, which function as cation-dependent cell adhesion molecules. They are heterodimers, formed from α and β subunits; their primary function is in the formation of interactions between the cell and macromolecules in the ECM, and is the most important receptors for ECM proteins, such as fibronectin, laminins, collagens or vitronectin (Rüegg et al., 2004). Integrin binding to extracellular ligands results in integrin clustering to form 'focal adhesion complexes' and resultant activation of integrin- regulated intercellular anti-apoptotic, pro-proliferative and pro-migratory pathways. Integrin expressions are altered in malignant cells as compared to their normal counterparts and are appeared to be involved in several aspects of tumour growth, invasion and metastasis (Giancotti and Mainiero, 1994). Integrins provide an anchorage for cells to the ECM and are involved in directed invasion and motility of cells (Curran and Murray, 2000). Investigations have shown that down-regulation of α3 integrin subunit may contribute to the enhanced tumourogenicity of c-myc- over expressing small cell lung carcinoma, while the loss of α_v expression is correlated with the recurrence in node-negative lung carcinoma (Guo and Giancotti, 2004, Thiery, 2002). Reduced $\alpha_3\beta_1$ integrin expression is probably related to the increased aggressiveness and a poor factor of prognosis in patients either with small cell lung cancer (SCLC) or non-small cell lung cancer (Gogali et al., 2004, Adachi et al., 1998). Studies have also shown altered expression of α_v integrins in breast and renal carcinomas (Pignatelli et al., 1992, Korhonen et al., 1992). The role of $\alpha_5\beta_1$ in inhibiting cell proliferation has also been demonstrated in erythroleukaemic cells (Symington, 1990). Integrins involved in tissue organization are decreased, while those that permit cellular migration are maintained or upregulated. For eg; the αvβ3 integrin is poorly expressed by normal cells but is upregulated in many invasive and metastatic cancers.

Immunoglobulin Superfamily

A number of cell adhesion molecules that share the basic architecture of the immunoglobulin, classifed as members of the immunoglobulin superfamily. They interact with homophilic binding and heterophilic interactions with a variety of diferent ligands and play major roles in determining embryonic and neural development, wound healing and inflammation (Meyer and Hart, 1998). The members bind between themselves and with integrins and ECM proteins. Immunoglobulin-like molecules were originally designated as leukocyte-activating factor-1 ligands, but now they are better known as intercellular adhesion molecules (Serafini and Rosemurgy, 2000). Major members include Inter-Cellular Adhesion Molecule (ICAM-1, and ICAM-2), vascular cell adhesion molecule (V-CAM-1) and Platelet Endothelial Cell Adhesion Molecule (PECAM). During infammation, cytokines including TNFα and interleukin-1, induce the expression of such immunoglobulin family members as ICAM-1, ICAM-2, V-CAM and PECAM on the endothelial wall. These interact with a number of integrins expressed on the surface of leucocytes causing them to arrest prior to extravasation (Meyer and Hart, 1998). ICAM-1 also known as CD54 (Cluster of Differentiation 54) is not only an adhesion molecule but also a co-stimulatory molecule that provides signal to cytotoxic T lymphocytes (CTL) and natural killer (NK) cells (Van Seventer et al., 1990, Chong et al., 1994). Vascular cell adhesion protein 1 also known as vascular cell adhesion molecule 1 (VCAM-1) or cluster of differentiation 106 (CD106). VCAM-1 is expressed on activated human endothelial cells and is upregulated in response to tumour necrosis factor-alpha (TNF-alpha), interleukin-1 (IL-1) and lipopolysaccharide (LPS). It is involved in the adhesion of lymphocytes, monocytes and eosinophils to the vascular endothelium. It is upregulated on metastatic tumour cells, and it mediates the adhesion of melanoma cells to the endothelium (Bao et al., 1993, Rice and Bevilacqua, 1989). Certain melanoma cells can use VCAM-1 to adhere to the endothelium, and VCAM-1 may participate in monocyte recruitment to atherosclerotic sites. As a result, VCAM-1 is a potential drug target. ICAM-1 and VCAM-1 plays an important role in tumor angiogenesis and metastasis (O'hanlon et al., 2002). PECAM-1, also called cluster of differentiation molecule 31 (CD31). It plays a key role in removing aged neutrophils from the body. CD-31 is normally found on endothelial cells, platelets, macrophages and Kupffer cells, granulocytes, T/NK cells, lymphocytes, megakaryocytes, osteoclasts, neutrophils. Both PECAM-1 and another immunoglobulin superfamily member integrin-associated protein (IAP) are involved in leukocyte trans-endothelial migration (Lukas and Dvorak, 2004).

Other Adhesion Molecules

67-kDa Laminin Receptor

The 67-kDa laminin receptor (67LR) is a non-integrin cell-surface receptor with a high affinity for laminin. It has been reported that the 67-kDa laminin receptor (67LR) is implicated in cancer metastasis. Highly metastatic cells express significantly more 67-kDa laminin receptor on their surface. Expression is higher in most solid tumors. In colon and gastric cancer, there was a direct positive correlation between the expression of the 67-kDa receptor in the primary tumor and the metastatic potential of the lesion (Givant-Horwitz et al., 2004).

CD44

CD44 is a trans-membrane glycoprotein that binds extracellular matrix components such as such as hyaluronic acid, fibronectin, collagen and the pro-metastatic factor, osteopontin (Tokumo et al., 1998). CD44 is proposed to modulate adhesion, lymphocyte homing and activation (Lesley et al., 1993, Stafford et al., 2008). For tumour metastasis to occur through the blood vessel and lymphatic vessel pathway, the tumour cells must first adhere to endothelial cells.

Studies have shown that high expression of CD44 in certain types of tumours is associated with the hematogenic spread of cancer cells (Wang et al., 2005). In different human tumours, expression of CD44 is correlated with an advanced stage of tumour growth and metastatic potential and therefore reduces the long-term survival of patients (Dall et al., 1995).

Serum CD44 levels have also been suggested as indicators of tumor burden and metastatic spread, with 20 fold greater amounts of CD44 being detected in serum from gastric and colorectal carcinoma patients (Guo et al., 1994).

Tumour Cell Invasion

Tumour invasion is the active migration of neoplastic cells out of their tissue of origin and into adjacent tissues of different types. The process is completed in 3 steps. The first step is tumour cell attachment via cell surface receptors which specifically bind to components of the matrix such as laminin (for the basement membrane) and fibronectin (for the stroma). The anchored tumor cell next secretes hydrolytic enzymes (or induces host cells to secrete enzymes) which can locally degrade the matrix (including degradation of the attachment components). Matrix lysis most probably takes place in a highly localized region close to the tumour cell surface. The third step is tumour cell locomotion into the region of the matrix modified by proteolysis. An early step in locomotion is pseudopodial protrusion at the leading edge of the migrating cell. Continued invasion of the matrix may take place by cyclic repetition of these three steps (Liotta, 1986).

Attachment to ECM

The ability of tumour cells to form transient attachments is necessary for metastasis. Metastasizing tumour cells must be able to attach to extracellular matrix components and to other cells (of the same or different type).

ECM is mainly composed of several proteoglycans as co-receptors and proteins such as collagen, laminin, and fibronectin. Integrins may play a critical role in the attachment of tumour cells to the extracellular matrix (Danen et al., 1995).

Integrin-mediated signalling provides the most significant contribution to cell adhesion. Collagens are the most abundant protein constituents of ECM. Among these, type IV collagen is the major component of the basal lamina. Laminin binds to type IV collagen and the cell membrane as a structural component of all basement membranes, and mediates cell-matrix interactions to promote adhesion protein is involved in cell adhesion, growth, migration, and differentiation (Choi et al., 2010).

Degradation of ECM

In order for cells to migrate, they must be able to degrade the protein barriers. Degradation of basement membrane is a crucial event in invasion. Basement membranes and connective tissues consist of four major groups of molecules: collagens, elastin, glycoproteins, and proteoglycans. The quantity of each of these differs among basement membranes of different tissues.

These extracellular matrix constituents are stabilized and organized by various protein-protein and polysaccharide-protein interactions that can be destabilized by degradative enzymes (Fidler, 1991), generally called proteases.

Protease: Serine Protease, Cathepsins and MMPs

In cancer, altered proteolysis leads to unregulated tumour growth, tissue remodeling, inflammation, tissue invasion, and metastasis (Kessenbrock et al., 2010). Proteolysis of extracellular matrix (ECM) and basement membrane is an essential mechanism used by cancer cells for their invasion and metastasis. Many proteases are capable of degrading extracellular matrix components. Table 2 shows important classes of Proteinases (Castells and Rustgi, 2003). They are divided into three groups: Serine proteases, Cathepsins, and Matrix metalloproteases (MMPs).

Table 2. Proteinases

Serine proteinases
Urokinase plasminogen activator (uPA)
Tissue-type plasminogen activator (tPA)
Plasminogen
Plasmin
Thrombin
Elastase
Cathepsins
Cathepsin D
Cathepsin B
Cathepsin L
Matrix metalloproteinases (MMP)
MMP-1 (interstitial collagenase)
MMP-2 (type IV collagenase, gelatinase A)
MMP-3 (stromelysin-1)
MMP-7 (matrilysin, pump-7)
MMP-8 (neutrophil collagenase)
MMP-9 (type IV collagenase, gelatinase B)
MMP-10 (stromelysin-2)
MMP-11 (stromelysin-3)
MMP-12 (metalloelastase)

Urokinase plasminogen actvator (uPA) is the most important member of the serine protease family involved in ECM degradation. It is secreted as an inactive, single chain precursor that requires binding to its cell membrane receptor for activation (Neal and Berry, 2006). Members of this system, including uPA and its receptor (uPAR), are over expressed in several malignant tumours. This system plays a major role in adhesion, migration, invasion and metastasis of cancer cells, thus making it an important target for anticancer drug therapy (Mekkawy et al., 2009).

Upon binding to uPAR, pro-uPA is converted to its active form, which is then capable of cleaving plasminogen to plasmin. Plasmin can then degrade components of the basement membrane and extracellular matrix components including Fibronectin, Vitronectin, Laminin and Fibrin, a prerequisite for tumour cell invasion and metastasis (Blasi and Carmeliet, 2002). Plasmin also activates enzymes of the matrix metalloprotease family. The activity of uPA is regulated by Plasminogen activator inhibitors (type -1,-2,-3) and the protease nexin -1.

Matrix Metalloproteases (MMPs)

The matrix metalloproteinases (MMP) are a family of enzymes considered to be primarily responsible for extracellular matrix (ECM) degradation. These enzymes are secreted in inactive proenzymatic forms, are zinc-dependent, and can be subdivided on the basis of preferential extracellular matrix substrate (Kessenbrock et al., 2010). In particular, the MMPs include the only enzymes known to be capable of degrading fibrillar collagen (Curran and Murray, 2000).

Matrix metalloproteinases are secreted as proenzymes that require extracellular activation. They are divided into five general classes: (1) interstitial collagenases, (2) stromelysins, (3) gelatinases (type IV collagenases), (4) matrilysins and (5) Membrane-type MMPs.

MMP-2 and MMP-9 are the most important gelatinases involved in the basement membrane collagen IV degradation. MMP-2 (72 kDa) also called gelatinase A, constitutively expressed by most cells including endothelial and epithelial cells. The 92 kDa MMP-9 (gelatinase B) is produced by inflammatory cells, including blood neutrophils and tissue macrophages, as well as by stimulated connective tissue cells. MMP-2 is secreted as an inactive pro-form; when it is converted to a 62 kDa active form it can degrade collagen types IV and V, laminin and elastin. Membrane-type matrix metalloproteinase (MT1-MMP) that appears to be important in cellular activation of MMP-2 (Foda and Zucker, 2001). A positive correlation between tumour progression and the expression of MMP-2 and MMP-9 in tumour tissues has been demonstrated in numerous human and animal studies. Metastatic cells produce specialised cell-surface structures called invadopodia, which utilize proteases to degrade ECM components such as fibronectin, laminin, type I and IV collagens etc.

Regulation of MMPs

MMP activity is regulated at three levels: transcription, proteolytic activation of the zymogen and inhibition of the active enzyme. MMPs are expressed in tissues at various stages of development but are typically absent in normal cells of the adult organism (Stamenkovic, 2000). MMPs can be activated by various external stimuli, including cytokines, growth factors and changes in cell–cell and cell–ECM interactions.

MMP expression is primarily regulated at the transcriptional level, which is regulated either positively or negatively by cytokines and growth factors such as interleukins (IL-1, IL-4, and IL-6), transforming growth factors (EGF, HGF, and TGFβ), or tumor necrosis factor alpha (TNFα) (Kupai et al., 2010). MMPs are generally expressed in very low amounts in latent forms (Pro-MMP). Generally MMPs are kept inactive by interaction between cystein-sulphohydryl group in pro-peptide domain and the Zn^+ bound to catalytic domain. Activation requires the proteolytic removal of pro-peptide domain, mechanism of activation is called "cystein switch". Serine proteinase, plasmin has been observed to proteolytically activate a number of latent MMPs (Kessenbrock et al., 2010).

Tissue Inhibitors of Metalloproteinases (TIMPs)

The proteolytic activity of MMPs is primarily controlled by its natural inhibitors, Tissue inhibitors of metalloproteinases (TIMPs). They are consequently important regulators of ECM turnover, tissue remodeling and cellular behaviour (Brew and Nagase, 2010). TIMPs are small proteins of 21–

28 kDa that specifically block MMP activity by binding to the highly conserved zinc-binding site of active MMPs. There is balance between the levels of activated MMPs and TIMPs in normal cells and altering this equilibrium affects the process of cellular invasion.

There are currently four known TIMP family members. TIMP-1, TIMP-2, TIMP-3 and TIMP-4. TIMP-1 and TIMP-2 inhibit the activity of most MMPs. TIMP-1 can form a complex with pro-MMP-9, similarly TIMP-2 with pro-MMP-2 (Stamenkovic, 2000). Increased TIMP-1 and TIMP-2 levels in human cancer tissues have been associated with poor prognoses (Foda and Zucker, 2001). Numerous studies correlate low TlMP expression with enhanced invasive and metastatic properties in a number of murine and human tumour cell lines. Therefore, TlMPs play a critical role in the regulation of tissue degradation in metastatic diseases, but their use as pharmacologic inhibitors of MMPs has been limited due to the short half-life of the TIMPs, when administered *in vivo* (Ray and Stetler-Stevenson, 1994).

Migration

In order for cancer cells to spread to distant sites, they often must first migrate away from the primary tumour as part of the invasive process. Cell migration across exracellular matrix completed in a continuous cycle of interdependent steps. First, the moving cell becomes polarized and elongates. 1) Protrusion of the cell membrane forms pseudopodia that is mediated by actin polymerization, which attaches to the ECM substrate and 2) forms focal adhesion complex (FAK) 3) unactivated integrin subunits continually recycle along the cell surface 4) change in integrin affinity engages the ECM and a force is generated 5) the FAK is disrupted at the trailing edge of the cell 6) integrin complexes release (proteolytic disruption of FAK). During this cascade regions of the leading edge or the entire cell body contract, thereby generating traction force that leads to the gradual forward gliding of the cell body and its trailing edge (Gupta and Massagué, 2006). Numerous migration factors have been identified that appear to be associated with cancer cell migration (Oppenheimer, 2006). A series of proteins on the surface of the pseudopodia coordinate sensing, protrusion, burrowing, and traction. Proteinases at the pseudopodia tip may locally disrupt the extracellular matrix and permit forward extention (Kohn and Liotta, 1995) Tumor cells secrete factors that function as autocrine motility factors. Adhesion molecules play an essential role in tumour cell motility across the extracellular matrix. Cells cytoplasmic protrusions become tightly adherent at its tip. The $\alpha_3\beta_1$ and $\alpha_5\beta_1$ integrins play major organisation roles in the adhesion and formation of invadopodia promoting invasive cell behaviour (Lukas and Dvorak, 2004). Three types of tumour cell migration were characterized so far: mezenchymal, amoeboid and collective. In mezechymal and amoeboid types of tumour cell migration, cells move individually. Diverse types of tumour cell locomotion differ with cell protrusions and signalling pathways that control those processes (Popow-Wo niak et al., 2009).

Intravasation

For cancer cells to spread to distant organs they need to enter either the blood or lymphatic vasculature. Tumour cells enter into blood stream by digesting basement membrane. The mechanistic cascade is similar to invasion. Metastatic tumor cells first attach to the endothelial basement membrane, digest it by secreting powerful proteases, and migrate between the endothelial cells to enter the bloodstream. Entry into lymphatic vasculature is also an important route of tumour cell dissemination as the process is simpler due to the absence of a basement membrane.

Cancer Cells in the Blood Stream

It is true that the majority of disseminating tumour cells die rapidly in the circulation due to nonspecific factors such as hemodynamic forces. They undergo severe damage and a large fraction of them (over 90%) die within 24 hours after intravasation. Lack of adhesion substrates, collision with cellular components in the blood stream, passage through narrow capillaries, and contact with blood components are all believed to influence the viability of circulating tumour cells (Kawaguchi, 2005). Although most tumour cells are quickly destroyed within the bloodstream, it appears that the greater the number of cells released by a primary tumour, they travel in clusters, increases the possibility that at least one will survive. Host factors such as T-cell, natural killer (NK) cell, endothelial cells, and macrophage activity may destroy circulating tumour cells (Xie and Huang, 2003). Tumour cells are surrounded with blood cells such as lymphocytes and platelets, which mask the cancer cells from immune surveillance. By facilitating cell arrest and adhesion to the endothelium, platelets encourage metastasis. Serotonin and thrombospondin, both released by activated platelets, have been implicated in increasing the likelihood of metastasis of circulating tumour cells (Nash et al., 2002).

Extravasation

Escape of tumour cells from blood vessels into surrounding tissues is called extravasation. The process is very similar to intravasation. First tumour cells in the circulation attach to the endothelial cells and then onto the basement membrane. α4β1 integrins or tumour cell proteoglycans (carbohydrate side chains) on tumour cells facilitate the adhesion to endothelial vascular adhesion molecules. Tumour cells digest the basement membrane by secreting protease and move through it (Neal and Berry, 2006). Extravasation occur through several mechanisms. In first mechanism tumour cells infiltrate into perivascular tissues by their own movement (locomotion type extravasation). The second mechanism involves sequestration of tumor cells beneath vascular endothelial cells, where they are separated from the blood stream. Third mechanism is explosive extravasation of tumour emboli (Kawaguchi, 2005).

Implantation into Target Organ: Specificity of Metastasis

Organ-specific homing and colonization of cancer cells (Tissue tropism) are important and interesting features of metastasis. Tissue tropism depends on both the histology and the stage of cancer. Cancers, such as breast, metastasize to multiple sites, most commonly lung and bone tissue and with less frequency the liver and the adrenal glands. Prostate cancer preferentially spreads to bone. Patients with colorectal cancer, by contrast, often develop initial metastases in liver (Chambers et al., 2002). Stephen Paget, 1989 proposed a "seed and soil" hypothesis that site specific lodging patterns were due to the 'dependence of the seed (the cancer cell) on the soil (the secondary organ) (Paget, 1989). Several factors are thought to influence the site of cancer metastasis, and these include (1) the pattern and direction of blood flow from the primary tumour, (2) mechanical trapping of tumour cells at a secondary site by small capillary beds, (3) tumour cell adhesion at a secondary site by the expression of appropriate cell surface proteins, and finally, (4) the microenvironment of the secondary site, which can create a permissive site for metastatic colonization of tumour cells (Horak and Steeg, 2005). Carbohydrates on the cancer-cell surface bind to a specific receptor selectin on the endothelial cells. Different selectins recognise different carbohydrates on the cancer cell surface. Each cancer-cell type expresses a different set of carbohydrates on its surface, attracted to different selectin molecules. The specificity of these interactions account for the differential homing specificities of different types of cancer cells.

Tumour Angiogenesis

Tumours cannot grow beyond a size of approximately 1–2mm without neovascularization (Folkman, 1990). So angiogenesis, a crucial event in cancer metastasis, is the sprouting of new capillaries from existing blood vessels, consists of a complex cascade of events including endothelial cell–mediated degradation and invasion of the extracellular matrix, endothelial cell migration, proliferation, differentiation, basement membrane deposition, and the organization of endothelial cords into capillary structures (Soriano et al., 2004).

Angiogenesis is mediated by several pro-angiogenic molecules released by both tumour cells and host cells including endothelial cells, epithelial cells, mesothelial cells and leucocytes.

Among these vascular endothelial growth factor (VEGF or vascular permeability factor, vasculotropin), members of the fibroblast growth factor (FGF) family, interleukin-8 (IL-8), angiogenin, angiotropin, epidermal growth factor (EGF), fibrin, nicotinamide, plateletderived endothelial cell growth factor (PD-ECGF), platelet derived growth factor (PDGF), transforming growth factor- α (TGF-α), TGF-β, and tumour necrosis factor-α (TNF-α) are important regulators (Ellis and Fidler, 1996).

These pro-angiogenic factors bind to receptors on nearby blood vessels and induce the activation, proliferation and migration of endothelial cells towards the tumour. Stimuli for the production of pro-angiogenic mediators include hypoxia, cytokines and growth factors, as well as mutations in oncogenes and tumour suppressor genes (Neal and Berry, 2006). The integrin family of cell adhesion proteins mediates cell attachment to the extracellular matrix and promotes the survival, proliferation, and motility of ECs during angiogenesis (Varner, 1997).

Table 3. Pro- and anti-angiogenic factors

Angiogenic factors
Vascular endothelial growth factor (VEGF)
Fibroblasts growth factors (FGF)
Epidermal growth factor (EGF)
Platelet-activating factor
Platelet-derived epidermal growth factor
Platelet-derived growth factor (PDGF)
Placenta growth factor
Transforming growth factor (TGF-α and -β)
Hepatocyte growth factor (HGF)
Tumor necrosis factor-α
Insulin-like growth factor (IGF)
Angiogenin
Angiopoeitin-1
Granulocyte-macrophage colony-stimulating factor (GM-CSF)
Granulocyte colony-stimulating factor (G-CSF)
Interleukin-2
Interleukin-6
Interleukin-8
Prostaglandins E1, E2
Vascular integrin αvβ3 (vitaxin)
Matrix metalloproteinases (MMP)
Antiangiogenic factors
Angiostatin
Thrombospondin
Fibronectin
Endostatin
Interferon-α,β,γ
Interleukin-1
Interleukin-12
Angiopoetin-2
Tissue inhibitors of metalloproteinases (TIMP)
Platelet factor 4
Retinoic acid

The process of angiogenesis can be completed in four steps, similar to tumour cell invasion process: (1) proliferation of endothelial cells; (2) breakdown of the extracellular matrix; and (3) migration of endothelial cells (4) tube formation and structural reorganization. Under normal physiological conditions angiogenic mediators establish a balance between the local pro-angiogenic and antiangiogenic functions by the receptors on the surface of the endothelial cells.

In pathological states such as chronic inflammation and tumour growth, there is an imbalance between endogenous stimulator and inhibitor levels, leading to an "angiogenic switch" (Ribatti, 2009) and has been recognized as key in promoting the transition towards a clinically aggressive tumour and that promotes and facilitates ''neo-angiogenesis''. Table 3. Shows a list of selected regulatory factors associated with the angiogenic process (Dong et al., 2007).

VEGF

One of the most important pro-angiogenic factor in the angiogenesis process is vascular endothelial growth factor (VEGF), which regulates endothelial proliferation, permeability, and survival. Four isoforms of VEGF exist, that bind to three receptors VEGFR-1 (Flt-1), VEGFR-2 (Flk-1/KDR), and VEGFR-3 (Flt-4) that are found on the surface of endothelial cells (Shepherd and Sridhar, 2003). Under hypoxia, hypoxia inducible factor-1alpha (HIF1-α) transcription is upregulated which then activates VEGF transcription, promoting the formation of abnormal blood vessels (Mendoza et al., 2008). VEGF stimulates ECM degradation, proliferation, migration, and tube formation of endothelial cells. VEGF promotes endothelial cell proliferation via the activation of the MAPK pathway (Wong et al., 2009). It induce survival signalling pathway by up regulating phosphatidylinositol-3' kinase (PI3K)/Akt, ERK kinases and Bcl-2 and also by down regulating p53, p21, p16, p27, and proapoptotic protein Bax (Nor et al., 1999, Wong et al., 2009). High circulating levels of VEGF correlate with poor prognosis in various solid tumours(Poon et al., 2001).

Metastasis Suppressor Genes

Metastasis suppressor genes (MSGs) do not affect the growth of the primary tumour but significantly inhibit the steps in the metastatic cascade and reduce the formation of secondary tumour. Many MSGs inhibit tumour cell motility and invasion in the primary tumour. Other MSGs regulate tumour cell arrest, extravasation, survival and growth at the secondary. Twenty-three such genes have now been described in the literature and collectively make up the metastasis suppressor gene family.

The first metastasis suppressor, Nm23 (non-metastatic clone-23), was identified in 1988. Nm23-H1 has been shown to suppress metastasis in several cancer models such as melanoma, prostate, colon, breast and oral squamous cell carcinomas. Studies demonstrated that transfection of the nm23-H1 gene to murine melanoma cell lines can suppress their metastatic potential(Utrera-Barillas et al., HORAK et al., 2008). Transfection of *nm23* gene into highly metastatic K-1735 melanoma cells reduced their *in vivo* metastatic ability by 52% to 96%, with no effect on the primary tumour size (Leone et al., 1991).

KISS1 gene is a metastatic suppressor gene encodes for secreted polypeptides, known as kisspeptins. It was first characterized in 1996. Multiple kisspeptins have been described, including metastin, a 54 amino acid polypeptide, which binds to the G protein coupled receptor GPR54, and is believed to be a peptide responsible for metastasis suppression. Down regulation of any one of the kisspetins or its receptor (GPR54) has been correlated with a poor clinical prognosis and more aggressive metastasis in oesophageal, bladder, gastric, thyroid and breast cancer (HORAK et al., 2008). Studies revealed that KISS1 secretion is crucial for multiple organ metastasis suppression and for maintenance of disseminated cells in a dormant state (Nash et al., 2007). The loss of KISS1 and KISS1R gene expression is closely associated with lymph node metastasis (Ikeguchi et al., 2004).

KAI1 (also known as CD82) is a metastasis-suppressor gene for prostate and breast carcinomas. KAI1 expression is down-regulated during prostate and breast cancer progression (Dong et al., 1995; Yang et al., 1997). HB2 mammary epithelial cells that overexpressed KAI1 showed decreased migration *in vitro* in response to EGF, compared with control transfectants (Steeg, 2003). The metastasis-suppressor activity of KAI1 was demonstrated by transfecting it into AT6.1 cells. KAI1 expression decreased both the invasiveness and motility of cells *in vitro* (Dong et al., 1995). Breast Cancer Metastasis Suppressor–1 (BRMS1) gene transfection inhibited metastasis in both breast carcinoma and melanoma cell lines, with no effect on tumorigenicity (Steeg, 2003). BRMS1 suppression of metastasis was correlated with reduced colonization in soft agar (Samant et al., 2000). BRMS1 interacts with NF-κB and decreases transcriptional activity by deacetylation of RelA (Liu et al., 2006).

Hypoxia and Metastasis

Tumour cannot grow beyond 1-2 mm^3 without proper blood supply (Wachsberger et al., 2003). Hypoxia is an important pathophysiologic feature in the microenvironment of solid tumours, which is caused by the imbalance between oxygen supply and consumption (Peng and Chen, 2010). Oxygen plays an important role in the generation of free radicals by ionizing radiation and subsequent radiation induced free radical mediated cancer cell damage. In the absence of oxygen, more radiation damage is repaired; thereby the effect of radiation is compromised (Peng and Chen, 2010). Radiation therapy therefore rescues metastatic radiation resistant hypoxic cells from dying and hence increased the probability of hypoxia induced metastasis. Tumour hypoxia is an environmental stimulus that plays a key role in the development and cancer progression, and is one of the major causes of treatment failure in radiotherapy and chemotherapy in cancer patients. The hypoxic response is mainly mediated by hypoxia inducible factor-1 (HIF-1) composed of HIF-1α alpha and HIF-1β beta, which becomes active under low oxygen condition. HIF-1 is generally regarded as the master regulator of the hypoxia response and is known to regulate several genes involved in regulation of metabolism, tumour angiogenesis and metastasis (Yang and Wu, 2008, Semenza, 2003). In normoxia, HIF-1α is hydroxylated and targeted for ubiquitination and proteasomal degradation (Denko, 2008). In hypoxic conditions it translocates to the nucleus where it dimerises with HIF-1β and binds to hypoxia responsive elements and activates transcription (Azam et al., 2010). Expression of HIF-1α is upregulated in many human cancers and is associated with treatment failure (Koukourakis et al., 2006, Bos et al., 2003). Tissue hypoxia can induce a number of angiogenic factors that promote angiogenesis, such as VEGF, IL-8, angiogenin, FGF, and PDGF. HIF-1α can stimulate the expression of vascular endothelial growth factor (VEGF)(Tsiokas et al., 1995). VEGF plays a major role in physiological blood vessel formation and pathological angiogenesis in tumour growth (Ellis and Hicklin, 2008). Several studies demonstrated that many antiangiogenic drugs could overcome tumour hypoxia and improve tumour response to radiation therapy (Wachsberger et al., 2003).

NF-κB and Metastasis

Nuclear factor- κB (NF-κB) belonging to Rel family of proteins consists of five members, namely: p65 (RelA), RelB, c-Rel, p50/p105 (NF-κB1) and p52/p100 (NF- κB2), and exist as homo-or heterodimers bound to the I-κB family of proteins. These proteins contain 300 amino acids that share homology with the v-Rel oncoprotein, known as the Rel homology domain (RHD) that is responsible for DNA binding, dimerization to other NF-κB subunits, and nuclear translocation (Bakkar and Guttridge, 2010). Classical NF- κB is a dimer composed of a p50 (NF κB1) and p65 (RelA) subunit. In non-stimulated state, NF- κB is sequestered in the cytoplasm by a family of specific inhibitory proteins termed I κBs. In response to a variety of stimuli such as TNF-α or IL-1, viruses, genotoxic agents and ionizing radiation, the IκB molecules are phosphorylated by the IκB kinase complex (IKK) leading to their ubiquitination and degradation by the proteasome pathway. NF-κB dimers are subsequently released and free to translocate to the nucleus where they activate transcription of various target genes that promote tumour cell proliferation, survival, metastasis, inflammation, invasion, and angiogenesis (Baud and Karin, 2009). NF-κB can modulate the transcriptional activation of genes associated with cell proliferation, angiogenesis, metastasis, tumour promotion, inflammation and suppression of apoptosis. Aberrant NF-κB regulation has been observed in many cancers (Luqman and Pezzuto, 2010).Tumour cell proliferation can be blocked by regulating NF-κB pathway, which makes tumour cells more sensitive antitumor agents (Karin, 2006). Studies demonstrate the NF-κB mediated activation of transcription factor, hypoxia-inducible factor-1 α, which regulates the expression of genes such as VEGF and COX-2 (Rius et al., 2008). NF-κB is a direct modulator for HIF-1α (Van Uden et al., 2008). NF-κB signalling pathway can be activated by several pro-inflammatory cytokines such as TNF-α, IL-1β, IL-6 and tumour promoting genes like VEGF, and COX-2 (Kawai and Akira, 2007, Hagemann et al., 2009, Karin and Greten, 2005). Cellular stresses such as ionizing radiation and chemotherapeutic agents also activate NF-κB (Sethi and Aggarwal, 2006). NF-κB can regulate the activation of cytokines, adhesion molecules, angiogenic factors, and MMPs that all have been associated with tumour progression and metastasis(Coussens and Werb, 2002). Several studies demonstrate the positive correlation between NF-κB and tumour metastasis(Marcello and Lakita, 2005). Thus NF-κB is an ideal target for anticancer drug development.

NO and Metastasis

Nitric oxide (NO) is a free radical that is involved in the every aspect of cancer, from tumorigenesis to metastasis. NO is produced via enzymatic action on L-arginine, with NADPH (reduced nicotinamide adenine dinucleotide) and oxygen as cofactors, and L-citrulline as secondary product (Xu et al., 2002). There are four nitric oxide synthase enzymes involved in NO production: induced nitric oxide synthase (iNOS), endothelial NO synthase (eNOS), neural NO synthase (nNOS), and mitochondrial NOS. Several studies indicate that NO can modulate cancer-related events including nitro-oxidative stress, apoptosis, cell cycle, angiogenesis, invasion, and metastasis (Yang et al., 2009). Overexpression of iNOS in cancer tissues is associated with poor prognosis in cancer patients (Yasuda, 2008). NO causes DNA damage and direct cell death at high concentrations, whereas it exerts antiapoptotic effects on cells at low concentrations (Wink et al., 1998). A highly metastatic cell line produce higher amount of NO and this was correlated with increased invasiveness (Jadeski et al., 2000). There was a positive correlation between VEGF and nitrate/nitrite level in serum of breast cancer patients (Cokun et al., 2003). NO can modulate several steps in the metastatic cascade, including suppression of platelet aggregation, down-regulation of the expression of CAMs, such as VCAM and ICAM, and inhibition of angiogenesis (Gatti et al., 2004). It was shown that NO induces the expression of VEGF in human carcinoma cells (Chin et al., 1997). NO enhanced invasiveness of the human colorectal adenocarcinoma cell line, HRT-18 (Siegert et al., 2002). Cytokines including IFN- γ, TNF- α, and IL-1β have been reported to induce iNOS and promote production of a large amount of NO in malignant cells (Geller et al., 1993).

Apoptosis and Metastasis

Programmed cell death (apoptosis) is an essential building block for the normal development of any multicellular organism. Dysregulation of apoptosis has long been linked to the development of cancer. Defects in apoptosis can also acivate protooncogenes, promote tumour cell invasion and metastasis (Green and Evan, 2002, Reed, 2003). In general, apoptosis can be initiated in two ways: by an intrinsic pathway (mitochondria mediated) and extrinsic (death receptor mediated). Intrinsic pathway is under the control of the Bcl-2 family and initiated by the release of cytochrome c from mitochondria. Cytosolic cytochrome c together with apoptosis protease activating factor (Apaf)-1 activates caspase-9,which in turn activates effector caspases (eg: caspase-3) resulting in apoptosis. Extrinsic (death receptor-mediated) pathway is initiated by the interaction of the ligand with its death receptor, which leads to the activation of caspase-8 and -3. The caspase-3 then cleaves various substrates leading to apoptosis. Suppression of apoptosis promotes tumour metastasis. Most of the tumour cells that leave the primary tumour and enter the circulation die by apoptosis before they can establish secondary tumour. Bcl-2 overexpression led to a significantly higher rate of pulmonary metastasis (Bold et al., 1997). Reduced bcl-2 expression is associated with a lower probability of metastatic disease formation and longer survival in pancreatic cancer patients (Sinicrope et al., 1996). Highly metastatic cells exhibit superior survival ability and apoptosis resistance compared to poorly metastatic cells and also found that there was a genetic link between aggressive metastatic phenotype and apoptotic resistance (Glinsky and Glinsky, 1996).

p53 also called 'guardian of the genome', the first tumour suppressor gene involved in cell cycle regulation and induction of apoptosis. As a sensor of cellular stress, p53 is activated by a variety of stimuli such as anticancer drugs or irradiation, leading to cell cycle arrest and/or apoptosis (Vogelstein et al., 2000). Most of the human tumours are either p53 mutant or overexpressed with the antiapoptotic gene bcl-2 that enhances tumour cell proliferation and metastasis (Hainaut and Hollstein, 1999).

Bcl-2 family proteins are central regulators of the intrinsic pathway, which either suppress or promote changes in mitochondrial membrane permeability required for release of cyt-c and other apoptotic proteins (Reed, 2003). They comprises both proapoptotic and antiapoptotic members. Bcl-2, Bcl-XL and Bcl-w are anti apoptotic members inhibit apoptosis and promote cancer cell proliferation and metastasis. Proapoptotic members of the family include Bax, Bak, Bok and the BH3 subfamily comprising Bik, Bad, Bid, Bim, Noxa and Puma. Imbalances in the ratio of anti- and pro-apoptotic Bcl-2 proteins may favor tumor cell survival instead of cell death (Antonsson and Martinou, 2000). Overexpression of antiapoptotic genes were observed in more than half of all cancers, especially in highly metastatic cancers (Amundson et al., 2000).

Current Therapies

Treatments for metastatic cancer are currently similar to those used for primary tumours. Surgery is rarely performed on metastatic lesions. Radiation therapy and chemotherapy are major conventional treatment modalities. In radiation therapy high dose of X-rays damage the DNA of the cancerous tissue.

Chemotherapeutic agents destroy the cancer cells either directly or by inducing apoptosis. Some drugs halt cell division thereby preventing cancer cell proliferation. Immunomodulators are used to stimulate the body's defense mechanisms that effectively fight against cancer. In gene therapy cancer cells are genetically modified in such a way that immune system can easily recognize and attack them. Some cancers depend on hormones to grow, in such case, cancer growth is inhibited by regulating hormone production (Hormone therapy). Cancer vaccines are developed against tumor associated antigens (proteins). The immune system prepared to fight these antigens and go after these cells.

Therapeutic Targets

Based on the understanding of mechanisms underlying tumour invasion and metastasis, novel anticancer drugs are developed which can specifically target therapeutic sites. Some of the therapeutic targets and available drugs are as follows.

Angiogenesis: Vascularization of tumour tissue is essential for tumour progression and metastasis. Therefore inhibition of angiogenesis (the formation of new blood vessels) could play a crucial role in anti-metastatic therapy. Major angiogenic inhibitors are TNP-470 (AGM-1470) and, anti-vascular endothelial growth factor antibody (e.g. bevacizumab).

Motility: Cancer cell migration is essential for invasion and distant metastasis. Taxanes are the best example for motility inhibitor.

Matrix metalloproteinase: MMPs are upregulated in most of the human cancers. Hydroxamate molecules (Eg: Batimastat and marimastat) are the first class of MMP inhibitors which inhibit at the activation site, thus mimicking the physiologic action of TIMPs.

Vitronectin receptor integrin ($\alpha v\beta 3$): Antagonists of $\alpha v\beta 3$, LM609 and Vitaxin (monoclonal antibodies), induce vascular cell apoptosis and inhibit angiogenesis.

Conclusions

Tumour invasion and metastasis are the major challenges in the success of cancer therapy. Significant developments in the field of cancer research have made improvement in the diagnosis and treatment of various cancers. Primary cancer and its eradication are mainly based on surgery and radiation but these modalities produced only a little effect against metastatic cancers. But to some extent chemotherapy has made a promising effect in anti-metastatic therapy.

Metastasis involves a complex cascade of multiple tumour - host interactions contributing chemotherapeutic drug resistance. However, no drugs are presently available to specifically inhibit the metastasis of cancer cells. A better understanding of metastatic cascade and their molecular mechanism will leads to the invention of novel drug targets for therapeutic intervention in coming days.

Acknowledgment

The authors sincere thanking Dr. Ramadasan Kuttan, Research Director, Amala Cancer Research Centre, for his valuable suggestions.

References

Aberle, H., Schwartz, H. and Kemler, R. 1996. Cadherin-catenin complex: protein interactions and their implications for cadherin function. *Journal of cellular biochemistry,* 61, 514-523.

Adachi, M., Taki, T., Huang, C., Higashiyama, M., Doi, O., Tsuji, T. and Miyake, M. 1998. Reduced integrin alpha3 expression as a factor of poor prognosis of patients with adenocarcinoma of the lung. *Journal of Clinical Oncology,* 16, 1060.

Albelda, S. 1993. Role of integrins and other cell adhesion molecules in tumor progression and metastasis. *Laboratory investigation; a journal of technical methods and pathology,* 68, 4.

Amundson, S., Myers, T., Scudiero, D., Kitada, S., Reed, J. and Fornace, A. 2000. An informatics approach identifying markers of chemosensitivity in human cancer cell lines. *Cancer Research,* 60, 6101.

Antonsson, B. and Martinou, J. 2000. The Bcl-2 protein family. *Experimental Cell Research,* 256, 50.

Azam, F., Mehta, S. and Harris, A. 2010. Mechanisms of resistance to antiangiogenesis therapy. *European Journal of Cancer,* 46, 1323-1332.

Bakkar, N. and Guttridge, D. 2010. NF-{kappa} B Signaling: A Tale of Two Pathways in Skeletal Myogenesis. *Physiological reviews,* 90, 495.

Bao, L., Pigott, R., Matsumura, Y., Baban, D. and Tarin, D. 1993. Correlation of VLA-4 integrin expression with metastatic potential in various human tumour cell lines. *Differentiation,* 52, 239-246.

Baud, V. and Karin, M. 2009. Is NF- B a good target for cancer therapy? Hopes and pitfalls. *Nature Reviews Drug Discovery,* 8, 33-40.

Blasi, F. and Carmeliet, P. 2002. uPAR: a versatile signalling orchestrator. *Nature Reviews Molecular Cell Biology,* 3, 932-943.

Bold, R., Termuhlen, P. and McConkey, D. 1997. Apoptosis, cancer and cancer therapy. *Surgical oncology,* 6, 133-142.

Bos, R., van der Groep, P., Greijer, A., Shvarts, A., Meijer, S., Pinedo, H., Semenza, G., van Diest, P. and van der Wall, E. 2003. Levels of hypoxia inducible factor 1 independently predict prognosis in patients with lymph node negative breast carcinoma. *Cancer,* 97, 1573-1581.

Bremnes, R., Veve, R., Hirsch, F. and Franklin, W. 2002. The E-cadherin cell-cell adhesion complex and lung cancer invasion, metastasis, and prognosis. *Lung Cancer,* 36, 115-124.

Brew, K. and Nagase, H. 2010. The tissue inhibitors of metalloproteinases (TIMPs): An ancient family with structural and functional diversity. *Biochimica et Biophysica Acta (BBA)-Molecular Cell Research,* 1803, 55-71.

Castells, A. and Rustgi, A. K. 2003. Tumor Invasion and Metastasis. In: RUSTGI, A. K. and CRAWFORD, J. M. (Eds.) *Gastrointestinal cancers: a companion to Sleisenger and Fordtran's gastrointestinal and liver disease.* Philadelphia, Saunders.

Cavallaro, U. and Christofori, G. 2001. Cell adhesion in tumor invasion and metastasis: loss of the glue is not enough. *Biochim Biophys Acta,* 1552, 39-45.

Chambers, A., Groom, A. and MacDonald, I. 2002. Metastasis: dissemination and growth of cancer cells in metastatic sites. *Nature Reviews Cancer,* 2, 563-572.

Chin, K., Kurashima, Y., Ogura, T., Tajiri, H., Yoshida, S. and Esumi, H. 1997. Induction of vascular endothelial growth factor by nitric oxide in human glioblastoma and hepatocellular carcinoma cells. *Oncogene,* 15, 437.

Choi, B., Choi, Y., Kang, D., Kim, B., Song, Y. and Cha, H. 2010. Cell behavior on extracellular matrix mimic materials based on mussel adhesive protein fused with functional peptides. *Biomaterials,* 31, 0e8988.

Chong, A., Boussy, I., Jiang, X., Lamas, M. and Graf, L. 1994. CD54/ICAM-1 is a costimulator of NK cell-mediated cytotoxicity. *Cellular immunology,* 157, 92-105.

Cokun, U., Günel, N., Sancak, B., Günel, U., Onuk, E., Bayram, O., Yílmaz, E., Candan, S. and Ozkan, S. 2003. Significance of serum vascular endothelial growth factor, insulin-like growth factor-I levels and nitric oxide activity in breast cancer patients. *The Breast,* 12, 104-110.

Coman, D. 1944. Decreased mutual adhesiveness, a property of cells from squamous cell carcinomas. *Cancer Research,* 4, 625.

Coman, D. 1953. Mechanisms responsible for the origin and distribution of blood-borne tumor metastases: a review. *Cancer Research,* 13, 397.

Coussens, L. and Werb, Z. 2002. Inflammation and cancer. *Nature,* 420, 860-867.

Curran, S. and Murray, G. 2000. Matrix metalloproteinases:: molecular aspects of their roles in tumour invasion and metastasis. *European Journal of Cancer,* 36, 1621-1630.

Dall, P., Heider, K., Sinn, H., Skroch-Angel, P., Adolf, G., Kaufmann, M., Herrlich, P. and Ponta, H. 1995. Comparison of immunohistochemistry and RT-PCR for detection of CD44v-expression, a new prognostic factor in human breast cancer. *International Journal of Cancer,* 60, 471-477.

Danen, E., Van Muijen, G. and Ruiter, D. 1995. Role of integrins as signal transducing cell adhesion molecules in human cutaneous melanoma. *Cancer surveys,* 24, 43.

Denko, N. 2008. Hypoxia, HIF1 and glucose metabolism in the solid tumour. *Nature Reviews Cancer,* 8, 705-713.

Dong, J., Lamb, P., Rinker-Schaeffer, C., Vukanovic, J., Ichikawa, T., Isaacs, J. and Barrett, J. 1995. KAI1, a metastasis suppressor gene for prostate cancer on human chromosome 11p11. 2. *Science,* 268, 884.

Dong, X., Han, Z. and Yang, R. 2007. Angiogenesis and antiangiogenic therapy in hematologic malignancies. *Critical reviews in oncology/hematology,* 62, 105-118.

Ellis, L. and Fidler, I. 1996. Angiogenesis and metastasis. *European journal of cancer (Oxford, England: 1990),* 32, 2451.

Ellis, L. and Hicklin, D. 2008. VEGF-targeted therapy: mechanisms of anti-tumour activity. *Nature Reviews Cancer,* 8, 579-591.

Fidler, I. 1991. Cancer metastasis. *British medical bulletin,* 47, 157.

Foda, H. and Zucker, S. 2001. Matrix metalloproteinases in cancer invasion, metastasis and angiogenesis. *Drug discovery today,* 6, 478-482.

Folkman, J. 1990. What is the evidence that tumors are angiogenesis dependent? *Journal of the National Cancer Institute,* 82, 4.

Francavilla, C., Maddaluno, L. and Cavallaro, U. 2009. The functional role of cell adhesion molecules in tumor angiogenesis.), Elsevier.

Gatti, G., Simsek, S., Zurrida, S., Kurne, A., Giannetti, I., Demirer, S., Smeets, A., Caldarella, P., Vento, A. and Giraldo, A. 2004. Possible role of nitric oxide in the biology of breast carcinoma: review of the available literature. *The Breast,* 13, 1-6.

Geller, D., Nussler, A., Di Silvio, M., Lowenstein, C., Shapiro, R., Wang, S., Simmons, R. and Billiar, T. 1993. Cytokines, endotoxin, and glucocorticoids regulate the expression of inducible nitric oxide synthase in hepatocytes. *Proceedings of the National Academy of Sciences of the United States of America,* 90, 522.

Giancotti, F. and Mainiero, F. 1994. Integrin-mediated adhesion and signaling in tumorigenesis. *Biochimica et biophysica acta, CR. Reviews on cancer,* 1198, 47-64.

Givant-Horwitz, V., Davidson, B. and Reich, R. 2004. Laminin-induced signaling in tumor cells: The role of the Mr67, 000 laminin receptor. *Cancer Research,* 64, 3572-3579.

Glinsky, G. and Glinsky, V. 1996. Apoptosis and metastasis: a superior resistance of metastatic cancer cells to programmed cell death. *Cancer letters,* 101, 43-51.

Gogali, A., Charalabopoulos, K. and Constantopoulos, S. 2004. Integrin receptors in primary lung cancer. *Exp Oncol,* 26, 106-10.

Green, D. and Evan, G. 2002. A matter of life and death. *Cancer cell,* 1, 19-30.

Guo, W. and Giancotti, F. 2004. Integrin signalling during tumour progression. *Nature Reviews Molecular Cell Biology,* 5, 816-826.

Guo, Y., Liu, G., Wang, X., Jin, D., Wu, M., Ma, J. and Sy, M. 1994. Potential use of soluble CD44 in serum as indicator of tumor burden and metastasis in patients with gastric or colon cancer. *Cancer Research,* 54, 422.

Gupta, G. and Massagué, J. 2006. Cancer metastasis: building a framework. *Cell,* 127, 679-695.

Hagemann, T., Biswas, S., Lawrence, T., Sica, A. and Lewis, C. 2009. Regulation of macrophage function in tumors: the multifaceted role of NF-{kappa} B. *Blood,* 113, 3139.

Hainaut, P. and Hollstein, M. 1999. p53 and human cancer: the first ten thousand mutations. *Advances in cancer research,* 77, 81-86.

Horak, C., Lee, J., Marshall, J., Shreeve, S. and Steeg, P. 2008. The role of metastasis suppressor genes in metastatic dormancy. *APMIS,* 116, 586-601.

Horak, C. and Steeg, P. 2005. Metastasis gets site specific. *Cancer cell,* 8, 93-95.

Ikeguchi, M., Yamaguchi, K. and Kaibara, N. 2004. Clinical Significance of the Loss of KiSS-1 and Orphan G-Protein–Coupled Receptor (hOT7T175) Gene Expression in Esophageal Squamous Cell Carcinoma. *Clinical Cancer Research,* 10, 1379.

Jadeski, L., Hum, K., Chakraborty, C. and Lala, P. 2000. Nitric oxide promotes murine mammary tumour growth and metastasis by stimulating tumour cell migration, invasiveness and angiogenesis. *International Journal of Cancer,* 86, 30-39.

Karin, M. 2006. Nuclear factor- B in cancer development and progression. *Nature,* 441, 431-436.

Karin, M. and Greten, F. 2005. NF- B: linking inflammation and immunity to cancer development and progression. *Nature Reviews Immunology,* 5, 749-759.

Kashima, T., Nakamura, K., Kawaguchi, J., Takanashi, M., Ishida, T., Aburatani, H., Kudo, A., Fukayama, M. and Grigoriadis, A. 2003. Overexpression of cadherins suppresses pulmonary metastasis of osteosarcoma in vivo. *International Journal of Cancer,* 104, 147-154.

Kawaguchi, T. 2005. Cancer metastasis: characterization and identification of the behavior of metastatic tumor cells and the cell adhesion molecules, including carbohydrates. *Current Drug Targets-Cardiovascular and# 38; Hematological Disorders,* 5, 39-64.

Kawai, T. and Akira, S. 2007. Signaling to NF-[kappa] B by Toll-like receptors. *Trends in molecular medicine,* 13, 460-469.

Kessenbrock, K., Plaks, V. and Werb, Z. 2010. Matrix metalloproteinases: regulators of the tumor microenvironment. *Cell,* 141, 52-67.

Kohn, E. and Liotta, L. 1995. Molecular insights into cancer invasion: strategies for prevention and intervention. *Cancer Research,* 55, 1856.

Korhonen, M., Laitinen, L., Ylänne, J., Koukoulis, G., Quaranta, V., Juusela, H., Gould, V. and Virtanen, I. 1992. Integrin distributions in renal cell carcinomas of various grades of malignancy. *The American journal of pathology,* 141, 1161.

Koukourakis, M., Bentzen, S., Giatromanolaki, A., Wilson, G., Daley, F., Saunders, M., Dische, S., Sivridis, E. and Harris, A. 2006. Endogenous markers of two separate hypoxia response pathways (hypoxia inducible factor 2 alpha and carbonic anhydrase 9) are associated with radiotherapy failure in head and neck cancer patients recruited in the CHART randomized trial. *Journal of Clinical Oncology,* 24, 727.

Kupai, K., Szucs, G., Cseh, S., Hajdu, I., Csonka, C., Csont, T. and Ferdinandy, P. 2010. Matrix metalloproteinase activity assays: Importance of zymography. *Journal of pharmacological and toxicological methods,* 61, 205-209.

Leone, A., Flatow, U., King, C., Sandeen, M., Margulies, I., Liotta, L. and Steeg, P. 1991. Reduced tumor incidence, metastatic potential, and cytokine responsiveness of nm23-transfected melanoma cells. *Cell,* 65, 25.

Lesley, J., Hyman, R. and Kincade, P. 1993. CD44 and its interaction with extracellular matrix. *Advances in Immunology,* 54, 271-335.

Liotta, L. 1986. Tumor invasion and metastases—role of the extracellular matrix: Rhoads Memorial Award lecture. *Cancer Research,* 46, 1.

Liu, Y., Smith, P. and Jones, D. 2006. Breast cancer metastasis suppressor 1 functions as a corepressor by enhancing histone deacetylase 1-mediated deacetylation of RelA/p65 and promoting apoptosis. *Molecular and cellular biology,* 26, 8683.

Lukas, Z. and Dvorak, K. 2004. Adhesion molecules in biology and oncology. *Acta Vet Brno,* 73, 93-104.

Luqman, S. and Pezzuto, J. 2010. NF B: a promising target for natural products in cancer chemoprevention. *Phytotherapy Research,* 24, 949-963.

Marcello, A. and Lakita, G. C. 2005. Nuclear factor-κB and liver carcinogenesis. *Cancer letters,* 229, 157-169.

Mekkawy, A., Morris, D. and Pourgholami, M. 2009. Urokinase plasminogen activator system as a potential target for cancer therapy. *Future Oncol.,* 5, 1487-1499.

Mendoza, E., Burd, R., Wachsberger, P. and Dicker, A. 2008. Normalization of Tumor Vasculature and Improvement of Radiation Response by Antiangiogenic Agents. *Antiangiogenic Agents in Cancer Therapy*, 311-321.

Meyer, J. T., Thompson, P. M., Behringer, R., Steiner, R. C., Saxton, W. M. and Oppenheimer, S. B. 1983. Protease activity associated with loss of adhesiveness in mouse teratocarcinoma. *Exp. Cell Res.,* 143, 63-70.

Meyer, T. and Hart, I. 1998. Mechanisms of tumour metastasis. *European Journal of Cancer,* 34, 214-221.

Nash, G., Turner, L., Scully, M. and Kakkar, A. 2002. Platelets and cancer. *The Lancet Oncology,* 3, 425-430.

Nash, K., Phadke, P., Navenot, J., Hurst, D., Accavitti-Loper, M., Sztul, E., Vaidya, K., Frost, A., Kappes, J. and Peiper, S. 2007. Requirement of KISS1 secretion for multiple organ metastasis suppression and maintenance of tumor dormancy. *Journal of the National Cancer Institute,* 99, 309.

Neal, C. and Berry, D. 2006. Basic principles of the molecular biology of cancer II: angiogenesis, invasion and metastasis. *Surgery-Oxford-,* 24, 120.

Nor, J., Christensen, J., Mooney, D. and Polverini, P. 1999. Vascular endothelial growth factor (VEGF)-mediated angiogenesis is associated with enhanced endothelial cell survival and induction of Bcl-2 expression. *American Journal of Pathology,* 154, 375.

O'hanlon, D., Fitzsimons, H., Lynch, J., Tormey, S., Malone, C. and Given, H. 2002. Soluble adhesion molecules (E-selectin, ICAM-1 and VCAM-1) in breast carcinoma. *European Journal of Cancer,* 38, 2252-2257.

Okegawa, T., Pong, R., Li, Y. and Hsieh, J. 2004. The role of cell adhesion molecule in cancer progression and its application in cancer therapy. *Acta Biochimica Polonica-English Edition-,* 51, 445-458.

Oppenheimer, S. 2006. Cellular basis of cancer metastasis: A review of fundamentals and new advances. *Acta Histochemica,* 108, 327-334.

Oppenheimer, S. B., Edidin, M., Orr, C. W. and Roseman, S. 1969. An L-glutamine requirement for intercellular adhesion. *Proc. Natl. Acad. Sci. USA,* 63, 1395-402.

Paget, S. 1989. The distribution of secondary growths in cancer of the breast. 1889. *Cancer metastasis reviews,* 8, 98.

Palmieri, D., Chambers, A. F., Felding-Habermann, B., Huang, S. and Steeg, P. S. 2007. The biology of metastasis to a sanctuary site. *Clin. Cancer Res.,* 13, 1656-62.

Paschos, K., Canovas, D. and Bird, N. 2009. The role of cell adhesion molecules in the progression of colorectal cancer and the development of liver metastasis. *Cellular signalling,* 21, 665-674.

Peng, F. and Chen, M. 2010. Antiangiogenic therapy: a novel approach to overcome tumor hypoxia. *Chinese journal of cancer,* 29, 715.

Pignatelli, M., Cardillo, M., Hanby, A. and Stamp, G. 1992. Integrins and their accessory adhesion molecules in mammary carcinomas: loss of polarization in poorly differentiated tumors. *Human pathology,* 23, 1159-1166.

Poon, R., Fan, S. and Wong, J. 2001. Clinical implications of circulating angiogenic factors in cancer patients. *Journal of Clinical Oncology,* 19, 1207.

Popow-Wo niak, A., Nowak, D. and Malicka-B aszkiewicz, M. 2009. Types of tumor cells movement. *Postepy biochemii,* 55, 113.

Prodromou, C., Siligardi, G., O'Brien, R., Woolfson, D., Regan, L., Panaretou, B., Ladbury, J., Piper, P. and Pearl, L. 1999. Regulation of Hsp90 ATPase activity by tetratricopeptide repeat (TPR)-domain co-chaperones. *The EMBO Journal,* 18, 754-762.

Ramburan, A. and Govender, D. 2002. Cadherins and catenins in pathology. *Current Diagnostic Pathology,* 8, 305-317.

Ray, J. and Stetler-Stevenson, W. 1994. The role of matrix metalloproteases and their inhibitors in tumour invasion, metastasis and angiogenesis. *European Respiratory Journal,* 7, 2062.

Reed, J. 2003. Apoptosis-targeted therapies for cancer. *Cancer cell,* 3, 17.

Ribatti, D. 2009. Endogenous inhibitors of angiogenesis:: A historical review. *Leukemia research,* 33, 638-644.

Rice, G. and Bevilacqua, M. 1989. An inducible endothelial cell surface glycoprotein mediates melanoma adhesion. *Science,* 246, 1303.

Rius, J., Guma, M., Schachtrup, C., Akassoglou, K., Zinkernagel, A. S., Nizet, V., Johnson, R. S., Haddad, G. G. and Karin, M. 2008. NF-[kgr]B links innate immunity to the hypoxic response through transcriptional regulation of HIF-1[agr]. *Nature,* 453, 807-811.

Rüegg, C., Dormond, O. and Mariotti, A. 2004. Endothelial cell integrins and COX-2: mediators and therapeutic targets of tumor angiogenesis. *Biochimica et Biophysica Acta (BBA)-Reviews on Cancer,* 1654, 51-67.

Samant, R., Seraj, M., Saunders, M., Sakamaki, T., Shevde, L., Harms, J., Leonard, T., Goldberg, S., Budgeon, L. and Meehan, W. 2000. Analysis of mechanisms underlying BRMS1 suppression of metastasis. *Clinical and Experimental Metastasis,* 18, 683-693.

Semenza, G. 2003. Targeting HIF-1 for cancer therapy. *Nature Reviews Cancer,* 3, 721-732.

Serafini, F. and Rosemurgy, A. 2000. Adhesion molecules: clinical implications. *Surgery,* 127, 481.

Sethi, G. and Aggarwal, B. B. 2006. Role of NF-B and NF-B-regulated Gene Products in Chemoresistance and Radioresistance. *Current Cancer Therapy Reviews,* 2, 115-125.

Shepherd, F. and Sridhar, S. 2003. Angiogenesis inhibitors under study for the treatment of lung cancer. *Lung Cancer,* 41, 63-72.

Shiozaki, H., Oka, H., Inoue, M., Tamura, S. and Monden, M. 1996. E-cadherin mediated adhesion system in cancer cells. *Cancer,* 77, 1605-1613.

Siegert, A., Rosenberg, C., Schmitt, W., Denkert, C. and Hauptmann, S. 2002. Nitric oxide of human colorectal adenocarcinoma cell lines promotes tumour cell invasion. *British journal of cancer,* 86, 1310-1315.

Sinicrope, F., Evans, D., Leach, S., Cleary, K., Fenoglio, C., Lee, J. and Abbruzzese, J. 1996. bcl-2 and p53 expression in resectable pancreatic adenocarcinomas: association with clinical outcome. *Clinical Cancer Research,* 2, 2015.

Soriano, J., Liu, N., Gao, Y., Yao, Z., Ishibashi, T., Underhill, C., Burke, T. and Bottaro, D. 2004. Inhibition of angiogenesis by growth factor receptor bound protein 2-Src homology 2 domain bound antagonists. *Molecular cancer therapeutics,* 3, 1289.

Stafford, L., Vaidya, K. and Welch, D. 2008. Metastasis suppressors genes in cancer. *The International Journal of Biochemistry and Cell Biology,* 40, 874-891.

Stamenkovic, I. 2000. Matrix metalloproteinases in tumor invasion and metastasis.), Elsevier.

Starzinski-Powitz, A., Handrow-Metzmacher, H. and Kotzian, S. 1999. The putative role of cell adhesion molecules in endometriosis: can we learn from tumour metastasis? *Molecular medicine today,* 5, 304-309.

Steeg, P. 2003. Metastasis suppressors alter the signal transduction of cancer cells. *Nature Reviews Cancer,* 3, 55-63.

Symington, B. 1990. Fibronectin receptor overexpression and loss of transformed phenotype in a stable variant of the K562 cell line. *Cell Regulation,* 1, 637.

Thiery, J. 2002. Epithelial–mesenchymal transitions in tumour progression. *Nature Reviews Cancer,* 2, 442-454.

Thomas, G., Jones, J. and Speight, P. 1997. Integrins and oral cancer. *Oral oncology,* 33, 381-388.

Tokumo, K., Kodama, J., Seki, N., Miyagi, Y., Yoshinouchi, M. and Kudo, T. 1998. CD44 exon v6 correlates with cellular differentiation but not with progression and metastasis of cervical cancer. *European Journal of Cancer,* 34, 2107-2111.

Tselepis, C., Chidgey, M., North, A. and Garrod, D. 1998. Desmosomal adhesion inhibits invasive behavior. *Proceedings of the National Academy of Sciences of the United States of America,* 95, 8064.

Tsiokas, L., Mukhopadhyay, D. and Sukhatme, V. 1995. Hypoxic induction of human vascular endothelial growth factor expression through c-Src activation. *Nature,* 375, 15.

Utrera-Barillas, D., Salcedo-Vargas, M., Gariglio-Vidal, P., Hernandez-Hernandez, D., Gutierrez-Delgado, F. and Benitez-Bribiesca, L. H-ras and Nm23-H1 gene expression and proteolytic activity in squamous cell carcinoma of the uterine cervix. *Archives of medical research,* 31, 172.

Van Seventer, G., Shimizu, Y., Horgan, K. and Shaw, S. 1990. The LFA-1 ligand ICAM-1 provides an important costimulatory signal for T cell receptor-mediated activation of resting T cells. *The Journal of Immunology,* 144, 4579.

Van Uden, P., Kenneth, N. and Rocha, S. 2008. Regulation of hypoxia-inducible factor-1 by NF- B. *Biochemical Journal,* 412, 477.

Varner, J. 1997. The role of vascular cell integrins $\alpha_v\beta_3$ and $\alpha_v\beta_5$ in angiogenesis In: GOLDBERG, I. and ROSEN, E. (Eds.) *Regulation of Angiogenesis.* Switzerland, Birkhauser Verlag Basel.

Vogelstein, B., Lane, D. and Levine, A. 2000. Surfing the p53 network. *Nature,* 408, 307-310.

Wachsberger, P., Burd, R. and Dicker, A. 2003. Tumor response to ionizing radiation combined with antiangiogenesis or vascular targeting agents. *Clinical Cancer Research,* 9, 1957.

Wang, H., Hung, Y., Su, C., Peng, S., Guo, Y., Lai, M., Liu, C. and Hsu, J. 2005. CD44 Cross-linking induces integrin-mediated adhesion and transendothelial migration in breast cancer cell line by up-regulation of LFA-1 ([alpha] L [beta] 2) and VLA-4 ([alpha] 4 [beta] 1). *Experimental Cell Research,* 304, 116-126.

Wink, D., Vodovotz, Y., Laval, J., Laval, F., Dewhirst, M. and Mitchell, J. 1998. The multifaceted roles of nitric oxide in cancer. *Carcinogenesis,* 19, 711.

Wong, B., Rahmani, M., Luo, Z., Yanagawa, B., Wong, D., Luo, H. and McManus, B. 2009. Vascular Endothelial Growth Factor Increases Human Cardiac Microvascular Endothelial Cell Permeability to Low-Density Lipoproteins. *The Journal of heart and lung transplantation,* 28, 950-957.

Xie, K. and Huang, S. 2003. Contribution of nitric oxide-mediated apoptosis to cancer metastasis inefficiency* 1. *Free Radical Biology and Medicine,* 34, 969-986.

Xu, W., Liu, L., Loizidou, M., Ahmed, M. and Charles, I. 2002. The role of nitric oxide in cancer. *Cell research,* 12, 311.

Yang, G., Taboada, S. and Liao, J. 2009. Induced nitric oxide synthase as a major player in the oncogenic transformation of inflamed tissue. *Methods Mol. Biol.,* 512, 119-156.

Yang, M. and Wu, K. 2008. TWIST activation by hypoxia inducible factor-1 (HIF-1): implications in metastasis and development. *Cell cycle (Georgetown, Tex.),* 7, 2090.

Yasuda, H. 2008. Solid tumor physiology and hypoxia-induced chemo/radio-resistance: novel strategy for cancer therapy: nitric oxide donor as a therapeutic enhancer. *Nitric Oxide,* 19, 205-216.

In: Metastatic Melanoma
Editors: S.A. Klein and J.P. Beckler
ISBN 978-1-61209-915-6

Chapter III

Metastatic Melanoma in the Paediatric Age

Andrea Zangari,* Carmine Noviello and Rosella Tallarico
Paediatric Surgery Unit, Azienda Ospedali Riuniti di Ancona.
Umberto I – Lancisi, Salesi, Ancona, Italy

1. Paediatric Melanoma

Melanoma is a malignant tumour originating from melanocytes (cells responsible for generating melanin, the pigment that gives colour to skin, hair and eyes). This pigment is the strongest in moles. It is due to this reason that melanomas are usually brown or black in colour. Sometimes, melanomas stop producing the pigment and appear red, pink, and even skin-coloured.

Most of the reported cases of melanoma in children are cutaneous, noncutaneous cases (eye, unknown site) are rare. The most common site for melanoma in male is the upper back; in female, the most common sites are the lower legs and upper back.

Melanoma in children is rare. The annual incidence is 0.8 per million in the first decade of life: 2% of all reported melanomas have occurred in patients younger than 20 years, but only 0.3% to 0.4% of them have developed in

* Email: andreazangari@libero.it, Fax 0039 0715962379, Tel. 0039 0715962321, Mob. 0039 3496275540.

prepubertal age [1,2,3,4,5,6]. However, a profound change in the natural history of melanoma is occurring: it is much more frequent in children and teenagers (recently an increase in the incidence of melanoma in children was observed in some country such as in Australia [7] where the overall incidence of melanoma is 5 times that in Europe). A recent report from the Surveillance, Epidemiology, and End Results database confirms an increase in the incidence of melanoma in children of approximately 2.9% per year from 1973 to 2001 [8].

Skin pigmentation and environment (ultraviolet exposure, latitude) are important risk factors [9]: people with light skin, blue, gray, or green eyes, red or blond hair, and lots of freckles are at highest risk for developing melanoma. However it is generally accepted that the cause of melanoma is complex and includes family history of melanoma and melanoma susceptibility genes (CDKN2A and CDK4) [10,11]. Mutations in the gene CDKN2A within the 9p21 region have been demonstrated in familial melanoma kindreds. The CDKN2A gene is complex and codes for p16 and p14ARF, which both function to suppress cellular growth. An intact p16 inhibits cyclin-dependent kinases that promotes cellular proliferation by inhibiting the retinoblastoma protein. Therefore, an intact p16 is essential to arrest the cell cycle. The p14ARF may be important in enhancing the effect of another tumour suppressor, p53 [12].

The management of melanoma in children is debated because of a few cases reported by comparison with adults, moreover the majority of patients younger than 20 years are adolescents. In children the misdiagnosis of pigmented lesions is common (it has been reported in up to 40% of cases) and often leads to therapeutic delay [13].

Sometimes the clinical behaviour of melanoma in childhood is generally held to be the same as in adults although some data support an adverse prognostic role of younger age [14] and others suggest a better survival in children [1, 15, 16, 17].

Melanoma is a challenge even for clinicians who see pigmented skin lesions in children on a daily basis: benign lesions can have alarming melanoma-like features, whereas melanomas often have an atypical presentation as nodular, pedunculated, or amelanotic lesions, sometimes simulating pyogenic granulomas. Early signs of melanoma include the ABCDEs: asymmetry of lesion; border irregularity (bleeding or crusting); colour change or variegation (some lesions are amelanotic); diameter larger than 6 mm or growing lesion; evolving (surface changes, raised lesion, bleeding, crusting) or symptoms (itchiness or tenderness). The ABCD clinical rule (asymmetry, border irregularity, colour variability, diameter ≥6 mm) is useful and widely used in children as in adults, but some considerations are necessary: for example the size seems to be less important (benign nevi normally grow up to relatively large size as the child grows, whereas melanomas may be detected at a very small size).

Some data are important in paediatric age: about 1% to 2% of primary melanomas arise from mucous membrane melanocytes, approximately 5% to 10% of patients present with metastatic disease (usually in the lymph node basin) without an identifiable primary lesion and less than 2% of patients present with visceral metastases in the absence of a known primary lesion.

Regarding the development in a congenital nevus, the risk for developing melanoma in congenital nevi has been estimated to be between 2% and 20%, being higher for the giant forms and lower (0%–5%) for the small lesions [1, 18, 19].

Dysplastic nevi should also be considered potential precursors of melanoma. Some Authors report a tendency for thicker lesions and later stages in pediatric melanoma probably as a result of a delay in diagnosis or very rapid growth[18, 20].

The clinical presentation of childhood melanoma can be atypical (in the Italian series, approximately half of the cases were clinically amelanotic). Particular vigilance should be maintained in children who have risk factors for the development of malignant melanoma: patients with xeroderma pigmentosum, dysplastic nevus syndrome and giant congenital melanocytic nevus, children who are immunosuppressed, and those with congenital nevi undergoing change. The classification and description of melanoma in children and adolescents has been exceptionally well addressed in recent reviews [18, 21] that classifies the melanoma into the four major categories: (A) melanomas arising in congenital giant nevi, (B) melanomas arising in other nevi and de novo, (C) central nervous system melanomas, and (D) other presentations.

Congenital giant nevi occur in 1 in 1000 to 1 in 20,000 newborns and may involve a very large surface area (usually defined as measuring at least 20 cm in diameter). These nevi are brown to black, may have a verrucous or lobulated surface, and may be accompanied by "satellite" lesions. 30% of melanomas in children develop within congenital nevi, with half of these appearing within the first 3 years of life. Primary cutaneous melanoma comprises about 40% to 50% of melanomas in childhood. They commonly present with changes in an existing melanocytic nevus (increase in size, bleeding, colour change, subcutaneous mass, and/or pruritis) which may be accompanied by lymphadenopathy. A rare variant of nodular cutaneous melanoma - Spitzoid melanoma - has characteristics of the benign Spitz nevus and has been misdiagnosed as such. Spitz nevi occur mostly in children and young adults and appear as dome-shaped, smooth, red-tan lesions less than 6 mm in diameter, located mainly on the head, neck, and lower extremities. Small congenital melanocytic nevi of less than 2 cm in diameter are more common than giant nevi, occurring in about 1 % of newborns. There are no clear guidelines for management of small congenital nevi due to inadequate evidence to prove increased risk for malignant degeneration. In spite of this, some investigators recommend excision of these nevi at puberty, believing that the risk of future melanoma outweighs the dangers of local anaesthesia [22].

Atypical mole syndrome is one of the major risk factors for cutaneous melanoma [23]. Both familial (autosomal dominant transmission) and sporadic types have been described. The lifetime risk of melanoma increases to 100% when two or more family members have been diagnosed with melanoma. Atypical mole syndrome is characterized by the presence of greater than 100 melanocytic nevi which are heterogeneous, variegated in colour, and irregular. These nevi may have an unusual pattern of distribution (buttocks, dorsum of the foot, scalp, iris, conjunctiva, and choroid). Management requires close follow-up of the patient whether or not other family members have melanoma. Total body photographs, nevus counts, and total body examinations by a dermatologist are recommended, along with counseling to avoid solar exposure and to use sunscreens.

The development of excessive melanocytic nevi in children who have been treated with immunosuppressive drugs is of concern because the risk of melanoma is related to the duration of immunosuppression.

Approximately 5% of cutaneous cancers in patients with xeroderma pigmentosum are melanomas, with an incidence of 1 in 5,000,000 [24].

Neurocutaneous melanosis is a rare disorder that consists of large pigmented nevi of the skin (usually the scalp or posterior midline) associated with leptomeningeal melanosis or melanoma. It often occurs with neurological symptoms such as headache and ataxia. The clinical course is marked by rapid progression toward death, with typical symptoms of seizures, psychiatric disorders, and communicating hydrocephalus. The nevus of Ota (hyperpigmented nevus on the eyelid and adjacent skin with pigmentation of the episclera, sclera and choroids) is particularly associated with leptomeningeal melanoma, as are Dandy-Walker malformation and Sturge-Weber syndrome. Primary leptomeningeal melanoma is an aggressive Central Nervous System melanoma, occuring in 75% of cases without cutaneous pigmented lesions. Because of its rarity (220 reported cases), poor prognosis and absence of cutaneous pigmentation, detection is difficult unless there is a high index of suspicion [25].

Early diagnosis of malignant melanoma in children is dependent on recognition of the fact that this tumour occurs in children.

Some Authors [18] recommend that suspicious pigmented lesions undergo excisional biopsy to ensure early diagnosis and prompt surgery, but some others say that excision is useful in cases of well-founded clinical suspicion of malignancy [26]. Diagnostic criteria include the distinction from melamomas mimics: atypical nevi, Spitz tumours, and lesions presenting asymmetry, border notching, colour variegation, diameter of more than 5 mm, rapid onset or increase in diameter, as well as bleeding, ulceration, itching, and pain [27]. We believe that any pigmented lesion that develops an irregular border, a focal increase or decrease in pigmentation, an irregular topography or ulceration should be evaluated immediately by excisional biopsy.

Melanoma mortality rates in children and adolescents are considered to be comparable to those in adults, although delays in detection and treatment can result in deep invasion and metastases at time of diagnosis with a less favourable prognosis. Prompt identification of pediatric patients with melanoma should result in increased survival. It is clear that surgery is effective as the primary treatment for children based simply on the numerous case series reporting long-term survival in some patients.

Primary treatment of malignant melanoma in children is surgical. Excisional biopsy of a suspect lesion is at the same time diagnostic and the first step of surgical treatment. The biopsy should include the full thickness of the dermis to facilitate measurement of the depth of tissue invasion (measured from the granular layer of epidermis) if a malignancy is confirmed histologically. The depth of invasion of the primary tumour in children, as in adults, has been reported to correlate with prognosis. Once the diagnosis has been established surgical excision with adequate margins should be performed [27]. Surgery is the mainstay and the only effective therapy for primary lesions and for positive lymph nodes.

The use of interferon as an adjuvant treatment has been reported in children, but its effectiveness remains controversial. Chemotherapeutic agents and radiation did not prove efficacious in the treatment of disseminated melanoma. The inadequacy of secondary modalities for treatment of melanoma further underscores the necessity for early diagnosis and prompt surgical treatment of this disorder in children. The sentinel lymph node biopsy (SLNB) technique is now generally accepted as being a safe and accurate method for staging regional lymph nodes and establishing any need for elective nodal dissection. As in adults this technique should be recommended in children with primary melanomas > 0.75 to 1 mm in thickness. Medical treatment may be useful in the case of disseminated disease and pediatric patients could be included in adult therapeutic trails (eg, immunotherapy, immunochemotherapy, vaccinotherapy).

Familiarization with both common and uncommon presentations of melanoma can avert delays in treatment and produce more favourable outcomes in youthful patients. Dermatologists play a central role in early identification of children at risk and can institute frequent surveillance of melanocytic nevi with total body skin examination and photography. Education of young people at an early age about the dangers of sun exposure and the wisdom of daily use of sunscreens may stimulate the child to form good skin care habits that survive into adulthood. A comprehensive sun protection regimen that can apply to adults as well as children may be helpful in preventing nonmelanoma skin cancers as well as melanoma, photoaging of the skin and ocular damage. The preventive role of surgical excision of giant and medium size congenital nevi is advocated by many Authors, depending on appropriate timing and case by case evaluation of the lesion [27, 28]. Melanoma can be a survivable disease if detected and treated appropriately in its early stages. Prevention is still the best strategy: patient and family education, sun protection, and early excision of large congenital nevi.

2. Metastatic Melanoma in Children

2.1. Congenital Melanoma and Transplacental Metastases

Congenital melanoma as a result of placental transmission from a mother with metastatic melanoma is extremely rare, as shown by the relatively small number of cases reported. Present knowledge of this subject is based on case reports and systematic reviews that have been published recently and there has been no population-based investigation of melanomas that arose from metastasis of maternal melanoma to the fetus [29, 30, 31, 32].

Weber et al in 1930 reported the first case in which the placental transmission of malignant melanoma from mother to fetus was described [33]. Afterwards 2 other cases of transplacental metastasis of malignant melanoma to the fetus have been reported in the English medical literature [34, 35]. Only six cases have been documented at present study. Melanoma is however the most common malignancy secondarily to involve the placenta. The subsequent fetal risk of developing melanoma has been calculated at 22% when placental metastasis is identified.

Existing reports suggest that melanomas which are diagnosed in utero have a poor prognosis, with subsequent death from disease in most reported cases [31].

To date, metastatic disease transmission from fetus to mother have never been reported [30, 36].

2.2. LYMPH Node Metastases

After early excision and diagnosis of primary melanoma, evaluation of lymph nodes status is essential for prognostic and therapeutic implications. Staging of the disease is completed by pathologic detection of lymphatic involvement, which will determine the treatment. Comprehensive staging guidelines for paediatric and adolescent melanoma have not been established and basic information regarding the characteristics of the primary tumour is lacking. Most Authors advocated grouping patients into three broad categories: localised disease, nodal spread and distant metastases.

The American Joint Committee on Cancer (AJCC) provides a reproducible model on the natural history of melanoma and a detailed description of important prognostic variables that are predictive of clinical outcome. For localised disease, ulceration has been recognized as an important predictor of outcome and there is growing consideration in defining the significance of melanoma thickness. For nodal spread, new importance has been recognized to the number of lymph nodes involved, as well as the significance of in-transit or satellite metastases. Metastatic disease has better been characterized by including a description of the sites of metastases and the prognostic value of serum lactic dehydrogenase (LDH) [37]. Future trials including paediatric and adolescent melanoma patients should incorporate this new staging system to achieve a wider interpretation of results from institutions and patient populations. In addition, the routine use of sentinel lymph node biopsy (SLNB) for the staging of paediatric and adolescent melanoma is mandatory, in order to determine the prognostic and therapeutic value of this procedure in young patients and to compare these results with those reported in the adult literature [38].

Although in the adult literature the routine use of computed tomography (CT) of chest or abdomen to stage patients with apparently localised disease is not recommended [39], a study at St Jude Hospital identified clinically undetectable metastases in 25% of paediatric patients with thick localised melanomas or in patients with melanoma arising at an unknown primary site [40]. The routine use of magnetic resonance imaging (MRI) to detect brain metastases is not advocated. In the presence of localised disease <1.5 mm thick, investigations include a complete blood count, serum chemistries (liver function tests too), and a chest radiograph. Although positron emission tomography (PET) has emerged as a useful imaging modality in patients with melanoma, there are no published studies using PET imaging to stage paediatric melanoma [37].

2.2.1. Sentinel Lymph Nodes

Early primary excision of melanoma is the mainstay of definitive treatment of melanoma. Nonetheless, SLNB has been of revolutionary importance for the treatment of patients with melanoma. Detection of sentinel lymph node metastases, through its prognostic value, has led to identification of patients who do not need elective lymph node dissection (ELND) and in which the morbidity linked to this procedure can be avoided. The techniques of preoperative lymphoscintigraphy and SLNB have become the standard of care for staging adult patients after detection of a primary melanoma. Staging of intermediate-thickness (1.2 - 3.5 mm) primary melanomas according to the results of SLNB provides important prognostic information and identifies patients with nodal metastases whose survival can be improved by elective lymphadenectomy. Morton et al. recently indicated a staging and prognostic value of SLNB in adult patients [41]. Such prognostic information would also be particularly useful in pediatric patients. Yet, data are controversial, and Roka et al could not find a predictive value of sentinel lymph node (SLN) status for overall survival [42]. Independent from prognostic value, a negative SLNB spares those patients from morbidity which was associated with ELND (wound infections, permanent nerve injury, chronic lymphedema). Because of the low number of melanomas during the first decades of life, only small series describing this procedure in pediatric and adolescent patients are published. There is lack of long-term follow-up data for patients in this age group, and therefore, the prognostic and therapeutic value of SLNB in the pediatric population remains to be defined. However, recent reports on SLNB in paediatric series refer to technical feasibility and low complication rate of this procedure [43, 44, 45].

Although comprehensive guidelines for the appropriate staging and workup for children and adolescents with melanoma have not been established, SLNB as a routine staging procedure should be included into the surgical management of younger patients or at least is a useful adjunct in determining the treatment of melanoma. The indications for SLNB in pediatric and adolescent patients are based on the adult literature and include the presence of lesions thicker than 1 mm or the presence of ulceration or a Clark's level of invasion of IV or V in patients with lesion thickness of less than 1 mm.

The technique is the same as in adults and its use in the paediatric age is described by several Authors. Excision of the primary tumour is performed with 2 mm margins of normal skin. After diagnosis of melanoma, the patient undergoes SLNB for melanoma thickness ≥ 1 mm, along with wide excision of the tumour site with 2 cm margins and primary closure or skin graft. SLNB is performed using preoperative lymphoscintigraphy, intraoperative blue dye injection around the site of excision and hand-held gamma probe for radiolocalization [27, 46]. Technical details are described by Topar et al. with the useful adjunct of subcutaneous infusion anaesthesia (SIA), as the first reported use in the paediatric patient: one day before the operation, between 18.5 and 40 MBq of Tc-99m microcolloid is injected intradermally around the excisional scar. The drainage of the colloid is localized by detecting the radiation, and the location of the SLN is marked on the skin of the patient. The location of the SLN is checked with a handheld gamma probe before starting the operation. At the site of the highest activity, SIA is infiltrated. A flow- and volume-controlled infusion pump is used with an initial flow of 300 mL/h. After a few minutes, the 30-gauge needle can be substituted by larger needles, and an increased flow (up to 700 mL/h deep in the axilla) can be used; 0.2% SIA solutions containing 450 mL of Ringer solution, 50 mL of Lidocainhydrochloride 2%, and 0.5 mL of Epinephrin are used. The upper limit of 0.2% SIA solution is 3 mL/kg in patients with body weight less than 50 kg, for patients with greater than 50 kg, a maximum quantity of 400 mL of 0.2% SIA solution can be used. After instillation of SIA solution in the SLN region, the primary scar is anesthetized. Patent blue is additionally injected intradermally around the scar as standard procedure. SLNB is then accomplished with the help of repeated measurements with the handheld gamma probe. The SLN(s) is (are) removed, and the wound is closed [47]. Several studies report that pediatric melanoma will have metastatic disease in about half of cases [47, 48, 49]. In some patients with head and neck and trunk melanomas lymphoscintigraphy may identify 2 areas suggestive for positive

SLNs. Such challenging drainage patterns underscores the vital role of SLNB as a tool to guide surgery with these localizations [48].

A comparison between melanoma in adults and in patients younger than 21 years who underwent lymph node evaluation either by lymph node dissection or SLNB showed a higher rate of lymph node metastasis in the pediatric group (44%) as compared to the adult group (23.9%). However this difference was not found to have statistical significance due to the small sample size and no statistically significant difference in the 5-year and 10-year disease-free and survival rates between the pediatric and adult patients was demonstrated. In this series, pediatric patients who had either Stage I or Stage II showed a 94.4% 10-year survival, while patients with Stage III melanoma had a 60.1% 10-year survival [50].

2.2.2. Regional Lymph Nodes

Evidence of melanoma cells in SLNs after biopsy leads to a completion lymph node dissection of the draining basin, avoiding the morbidity related to this procedure in SLNB negative patients. Survival advantage of completion lymph node dissection in melanoma is unclear, and this is actively being investigated in the Sunbelt Melanoma Trial [51]. It may be that indication to completion lymph node dissection is not supported by sufficient knowledge of how melanoma spreads, and it could actually be considered to be systemically metastatic at that point [52]. In the experience reported by some Authors, the SLN is often the only positive lymph node in the draining basin [53].

However, some Authors, although the issue is continuously under debate, would advocate the application of completion lymphadenectomy to achieve a potentially better outcome [48].

In fact surgery for melanoma is considered to have a key the role not only for diagnosis and staging but also for the eradication of the disease [54]. In a large series of paediatric melanomas eighteen patients underwent SNLB, and 7 proceeded to undergo complete lymph node dissection (CLND) because of findings of metastatic disease to the SLN; two of these 7 had tumor-positive lymph nodes on pathologic analysis of the CLND specimen [55].

Similarly, the presence of metastases in regional lymph nodes after CLND has been diagnosed in 1 of 3 patients by some Authors and in 1 of 4 patients by others [27, 48].

2.2.3. Adjuvant Therapy in Lymphatic Disease

Consideration of systemic therapy after regional lymph nodes involvement by melanoma cells is under investigation. Unfortunately, most trials of adjuvant therapy for melanoma do not include paediatric patients and therefore treatment plans for children must be extrapolated from adult studies. Traditional chemotherapy regimens did not show significant activity against melanoma. Interferon alfa-2b is currently used for adjuvant therapy in high-risk melanoma after surgery and adult studies have shown an improvement in relapse-free survival and overall survival when compared with observation. Pappo and colleagues at St. Jude Children's Research Hospital reported the experience of treating pediatric melanoma with high dose interferon in patients less than 18 years of age with Stage III melanoma, primary tumor thickness of greater than 4 mm or having lymph node or in-transit metastases, but no distant metastasis. Patients were treated with interferon alfa-2b intravenously during a 4-week induction phase and subsequently by maintenance therapy with subcutaneous administration three times a week for 48 weeks. All patients had completed induction therapy, and nine had completed maintenance therapy at the time of publication. The most common serious toxicity was neutropenia. Four patients manifested toxicity during the induction phase, and 3 required dose reduction during the maintenance phase. They concluded that interferon alfa-2b could be used in pediatric melanoma patients with acceptable toxicity. The study was not controlled, and therefore no conclusions about efficacy of the treatment could be reached. In a report from Toronto the use of high dose interferon in pediatric melanoma patients with metastatic disease on SLNB was examined. 6 patients of 10 who underwent SLNB were found to have SLNs containing melanoma cells. All patients who had positive SLNs then underwent CLND. Although most of the patients did complete their therapy, almost all required alterations in dosage due to toxicity, resulting in myelosuppression or abnormal hepatic function tests; 10 of the 11 patients survived with a median follow-up of 26 months; one patient died with metastatic disease. Because of the rarity of melanoma in the pediatric population it is difficult to institute clinical trials to evaluate adjuvant therapies. Histologic and clinical similarities in adult and pediatric melanoma suggest it would likely be helpful to include children in adult therapeutic trials [49, 53].

2.3. Distant Metastases

Patients with deeply invasive melanoma have a high probability of developing distant metastases. After invading deeper into the skin (Stages 0, I and II) until it hits the lymph nodes (Stage III), then melanoma is able to circulate throughout the body and metastasize in distant locations (Stage IV): the lung is most commonly involved, followed by brain, liver, bone marrow, heart and intestine [56].

Size and depth of invasion of the primary melanoma are correlated with the occurrence of metastases [57, 58, 59], but some variables which affect the distributions of metastases and organophilic behavior of this tumors are unknown.

Frequently metastases involve several organs, rarely a single site (1% to 5% of cases) [56]. Due to the rarity of malignant melanoma in children, little is known about the incidence that seems to be underestimated: several autopsies showed that patients with distant metastases generally have extensive dissemination to multiple organs [56, 60].

Clinical presentation depends of site and organ involved, for example patients with brain localization present with signs and symptoms of increased intracranial pressure or focal symptoms even if sometimes brain metastases are asymptomatic.

The diagnostic workup must extend beyond standard physical examination and chest radiographs: sometimes this examination can been negative despite of pulmonary metastases [60]. Additional studies, such as determination of the serum alkaline phosphatase, serum LDH concentration (LDH might help detect occult metastases) [61, 62] and other body imaging techniques (tomographic gallium scanning [63], computed tomography, or magnetic resonance imaging) are necessary.

In any patient with distant metastases limited to a single or a few sites, surgery should be considered as an option. However, even isolated metastases in distant sites such as brain can occasionally be removed with long-term survival after surgery [64] in other cases temozolomide, because of its oral route of administration and its ability to cross the blood–brain barrier, is a potentially attractive chemotherapy agent for patients with unresectable metastatic malignant melanoma [65].

The role of interferon in the treatment of melanoma is evolving and needs further study.

Systemic chemotherapy is primarily used in patients with stage IV (distant metastases) melanoma. Dacarbazine remains the most active drug: the response rate is in the range of 10% to 20%, and patients with metastases in the skin, subcutaneous tissues, or lymph nodes respond most often.

The biologic therapy (treatment directed toward modulating or inducing the immune system against melanoma) has gathered considerable interest, in fact Interleukin-2 (IL-2) [66] as a single agent has been used in metastatic melanoma. Monoclonal antibody therapies are still experimental and may be useful in melanoma.

Isolated limb perfusion has been used for metastases of an extremity [67]: the limb is isolated from the systemic circulation with a tourniquet, a chemotherapeutic agent is infused by means of a pump oxygenator, and then the medication is removed from the limb.

Radiation therapy is used for palliation some cases as brain metastases, pain associated with bone metastases, and superficial skin and subcutaneous metastases.

In a large paediatric series reported by Aldrink at al. among 150 patients twenty-nine developed metastatic disease, of which 19 developed central nervous system metastases, 4 pulmonary, 3 subcutaneous nodules, 2 liver, 2 bone, 2 small bowel, 1 pancreas, 1 adrenal, and 1 ovarian metastasis. Eight had metastatic disease, but record information about the site was unavailable. 24 of these patients ultimately died of their disease during the study period. Fourteen patients underwent resection of metastatic disease. Two patients underwent enucleation for ocular melanomas. Ninety-nine patients received immunomodulatory therapy in the form of an autologous vaccine. Nine patients underwent additional systemic therapy as chemotherapy, interleukin-2, or radiation therapy after resection of their primary lesion and/or recurrences [55].

The prognosis for patients with distant metastases of melanoma is poor in children as in adults and it is influenced by many factors: the anatomic site of disease (important determinant of respectability), presence of one or more metastases, localization of the disease to a single resectable organ or anatomic system and the presence of an elevated serum lactate dehydrogenase (LDH). A high proportion of soft tissue and extraregional nodal metastases allowed successful resection, irrespective of whether they were solitary or multifocal. Pulmonary, abdominal visceral, and bone metastases were completely resectable in only 40% of the patients. Metastases in the brain and liver were the least favourable in terms of resectability and survival.

The 5-year Survival rate reported in paediatric series ranged between 58.8% and 87.5%. In the report by Aldrink et al. of the 150 patients follow-up, obtained in 140 (93%), ranged from 1 month to 34.5 years and overall survival was 84% [37, 55, 68, 69]

However, spontaneous regression has been documented in melanoma, even in patients with metastatic disease [70].

References

[1] Pappo AS, Kaste SC, Rao BN, et al. Childhood melanoma. In: Balch CM, Houghton AN, Sober AJ, et al, eds. Cutaneous Melanoma. 3rd ed. Philadelphia, PA: JB Lippincott; 1997: 175–186.

[2] Ruiz-Maldonado R, De La Luz Orozco-Covarrubias M. Malignant melanoma in children. *Arch. Dermatol.* 1997; 133: 363–371.

[3] Boddie AW Jr, Smith JL Jr, McBride CM. Malignant melanoma in children and young adults: effect of diagnostic criteria on staging and end results. *South Med. J.* 1978; 71:1074–1078.

[4] Bader JL, Li FP, Olmstead PM, et al. Childhood malignant melanoma: incidence and etiology. *Am. J. Pediatr. Hematol. Oncol.* 1985; 7: 34–345.

[5] Conti EMS, Cercato MC, Gatta G, et al. Childhood melanoma in Europe since 1978: a population-based survival study. *Eur. J. Cancer.* 2001; 37: 780–784.

[6] Saenz NC, Saenz-Badillos J, Busam K, et al. Childhood melanoma survival. *Cancer.* 1999; 85: 750–754.

[7] Whiteman D, Valery P, McWhirter W, et al. Incidence of cutaneous childhood melanoma in Queensland, Australia. *Int. J. Cancer.* 1995; 63: 765–768.

[8] Strouse JJ, Fears TR, Tucker MA, et al: Pediatric melanoma: Risk factor and survival analysis of the surveillance, epidemiology and end results database. *J. Clin. Oncol.* 23: 4735-4741, 2005.

[9] Bressac-de-Paillerets B, Avril MF, Chompret A, et al. Genetic and environmental factors in cutaneous malignant melanoma. *Biochimie.* 2002; 84: 67–74.

[10] Tucker MA, Fraser MC, Goldstein AM, et al. A natural history of melanomas and dysplastic nevi: an atlas of lesions in melanoma-prone families. *Cancer.* 2002; 94: 3192–3209.

[11] Tucker MA, Goldstein AM. Melanoma aetiology: where are we? *Oncogene.* 2003; 22: 3042–3052.

[12] Hensin Tsao. Update on familial cancer syndromes and the skin. *J. Am. Acad. Dermatol.* 42: 2000; 939-969.

[13] Spatz A, Ruiter D, Hardmeier T, et al. Melanoma in childhood: an EORTC-MCG multicenter study on the clinicopathological aspects. *Int. J. Cancer.* 1996; 4: 317–324.

[14] Sander B, Karlsson P, Rosdahl I, et al. Cutaneous malignant melanoma in Swedish children and teenagers 1973–1992: a clinico-pathological study of 130 cases. *Int. J. Cancer*. 1999; 80: 646–651.
[15] Conti EMS, Cercato MC, Gatta G, et al. Childhood melanoma in Europe since 1978: a population-based survival study. *Eur. J. Cancer*. 2001; 37: 780–784.
[16] Hamre MR, Chuba P, Bakhshi S, et al. Cutaneous melanoma in childhood and adolescence. *Pediatr. Hematol. Oncol*. 2002;19: 309–317.
[17] Schmid-Wendtner MH, Berking C, Baumert J, et al. Cutaneous melanoma in childhood and adolescence: an analysis of 36 patients. *J. Am. Acad. Dermatol*. 2002; 46: 874–879.
[18] Ceballos PI, Ruiz-Maldonado R, Mihm MC Jr. Melanoma in children. *N. Engl. J. Med.* 1995; 332: 656–662.
[19] Gibbs P, Moore A, Robinson W, et al. Pediatric melanoma: are recent advances in the management of adult melanoma relevant to the pediatric population? *J. Pediatr Hematol. Oncol.* 2000; 22: 428–432.
[20] Mones JM, Ackerman AB. Melanomas in prepubescent children: review comprehensively, critique historically, criteria diagnostically, and course biologically. *Am. J. Dermatopathol*. 2003; 25: 223–238.
[21] Williams ML, Pennclla R. Melanoma, melanocytic nevi, and other melanoma risk factors in children. *J. Pediatr.* 1994; 124: 833-844.
[22] Roth MF, Grant-Kels JM. Important melanocytic lesions in childhood and adolescence. *Pediatr. Clin. NA* 1991; 38: 791-804.
[23] Kaiig S, Bamhill RL. Mihm MC, et al. Melanoma risk in individuals with clinically atypical nevi. *Arch. Dermatol.* 1994; 130: 999-1001.
[24] Mehregan AH. Mehregan DA. Malignant melanoma in childhood. *Cancer* 1993; 71: 4096-4103.
[25] Reyes-Mugica M, Chou P, Byrd S, et al. Nevomelanocytic proliferations in the central nervous system of children. *Cancer* 1993; 72: 2277-2285.
[26] Ferrari A, Bono A, Baldi M et al. Does Melanoma Behave Differently in Younger Children Than in Adults? A Retrospective Study of 33 Cases of Childhood Melanoma From a Single. *Pediatrics* 2005; 115; 649-654.
[27] Zangari A, Bernardini ML, Tallarico R et al. Indications for excision of nevi and melanoma diagnosed in a pediatric surgical unit. *J. Pediatr Surg*. 2007; 42: 1412-6.
[28] Paradela S, Fernández-Torres R, Fonseca E. Controversial Issues in Congenital Nevi Actas Dermo-Sifiliográficas (English Edition), Volume 100, Issue 7, 2009, Pages 548-561.

[29] Wiggins CL, Berwick M, Bishop JA. Malignant Melanoma in Pregnancy. *Obstet. Gynecol. Clin. North Am*. 2005 Dec; 32 (4): 559-68.
[30] Richardson SK, Tannous ZS, Mihm MC Jr. Congenital and infantile melanoma: review of the literature and report of an uncommon variant, pigment-synthesizing melanoma. *J. Am. Acad. Dermatol.* 2002 Jul;47(1):77-90.
[31] Alexander A, Samlowski WE, Grossman D et Al. Metastatic melanoma in pregnancy: risk of transplacental metastases in the infant. *J. Clin. Oncol*. 2003 Jun 1; 21(11):2179-86.
[32] Baergen RN, Johnson D, Moore T, et al. Maternal melanoma metastatic to the placenta: a case report and review of the literature. *Arch. Pathol. Lab. Med.* 1997 May;121(5):508-11.
[33] Weber FP, Schwarz E, Hellenschmied R. Spontaneous inoculation of melanotic sarcoma from mother to foetus: report of a case. *Br. Med. J.* 1930 Mar 22;1(3611):537-539.
[34] Dargeon HW, Eversole J, Del Duca V. Malignant melanoma in an infant. *Cancer* 1950; 3: 299-306.
[35] Brodsky I, Baren M, Kahn SB, et al. Metastatic malignant melanoma from mother to fetus. *Cancer* 1965;18: 1048-54.
[36] Brenn T, McKee PH. Melanoma in children and adolescents. *Diagnostic Histopathology,* Vol 14, Issue 1, January 2008, Pages 18-27.
[37] Pappo AS: Melanoma in children and adolescents. *Eur. J. Cancer*. 2003 Dec; 39(18):2651-61.
[38] Kogut KA, Fleming M, Pappo AS, et al. Sentinel lymph node biopsy for melanoma in young children. *J. Pediatr. Surg.* 2000; 35: 965-6.
[39] Buzaid AC, Sandler AB, Mani S, et al. Role of computed tomography in the staging of primary melanoma. *J. Clin. Oncol.* 1993, 11, 638–643.
[40] Kaste SC, Pappo AS, Jenkins III JJ, et al. Malignant melanoma in children: imaging spectrum. *Pediatr. Radiol.* 1996, 26, 800–805.
[41] Morton DL, Thompson JF, Cochran AJ, et al, MSLT Group. Sentinel node biopsy or nodal observation in melanoma. *N. Engl. J. Med.* 2006; 355: 1307-17.
[42] Roka F, Kittler H, Cauzig P, et al. Sentinel node status in melanoma patients is not predictive for overall survival upon multivariate analysis. *Br. J. Cancer* 2005; 92: 662-7.
[43] Roaten JB, Partrick DA, Pearlman N, et al. Sentinel lymph node biopsy for melanoma and other melanocytic tumors in adolescents. *J. Pediatr. Surg.* 2005; 40: 232-5.

[44] Toro J, Ranieri JM, Havlik RJ, et al. Sentinel lymph node biopsy in children and adolescents with malignant melanoma. *J. Pediatr. Surg.* 2003; 38: 1063-75.

[45] Pacella SJ, Lowe L, Bradford C, et al. The utility of sentinel lymph node biopsy in head and neck melanoma in the pediatric population. *Plast. Reconstr. Surg.* 2003;112:1257-65.

[46] Butter A, Huib T, Chapdelaine J, et al. Melanoma in children and the use of sentinel lymph node biopsy. *Journal of Pediatric Surgery* (2005) 40, 797–800.

[47] Topar G, Zelger B. Assessment of value of the sentinel lymph node biopsy in melanoma in children and adolescents and applicability of subcutaneous infusion anesthesia. *J. Pediatr. Surg.* 2007 Oct; 42 (10): 1716-20.

[48] Gow KW, Rapkin LB, Olson TA, et al. Sentinel lymph node biopsy in the pediatric population. *J. Pediatr. Surg.* 2008 Dec; 43 (12): 2193-8.

[49] Shah NC, Gerstle JT, Stuart M, et al. Use of sentinel lymph node biopsy and high-dose interferon in pediatric patients with high-risk melanoma: the Hospital for Sick Children experience. *J. Pediatr. Hematol. Oncol.* 2006; 28: 496-500.

[50] Livestro DP, Kaine EM, Michaelson JS, et al. Melanoma in the young: differences and similarities with adult melanoma: a case-matched controlled analysis. *Cancer* 2007; 110: 614–24.

[51] McMasters KM, Reintgen DS, Ross MI, et al. Sentinel lymph node biopsy for melanoma: controversy despite widespread agreement. *Journal of Clinical Oncology* 2001; 19: 2851–5.

[52] Pharis DB. Cutaneous melanoma: therapeutic lymph node and elective lymph node dissections, lymphatic mapping, and sentinel lymph node biopsy. *Dermatologic Therapy* 2005; 18: 397–406.

[53] Downard CD, Rapkin LB, Gow KW. Melanoma in children and adolescents. *Surg. Oncol.* 2007 Nov; 16 (3): 215-20.

[54] Sabel MS, Arora A. The role of the surgeon in the management of melanoma. *Minerva Chir.* 2006; 61: 54-141.

[55] Aldrink JH, Selim MA, Diesen DL, Johnson J, Pruitt SK, Tyler DS, Seigler HF: Pediatric melanoma: a single-institution experience of 150 patients. *J. Pediatr. Surg.* 2009 Aug;44(8):1514-21.

[56] Patel J K, Didolkar MS, Pickren JW, et al. Metastatic pattern of malignant melanoma. A study of 216 autopsy cases. *Am. J. Surg.*, 735: 807-810. 1978.

[57] Clark WH, Jr, Ainsworth AM, Bernardino EA, et al. The developmental biology of primary human malignant melanomas. *Semin. Oncol.*, 2: 83-103,1975.

[58] Lehman JA, Jr, Cross FS, Richey WG. Clinical study of forty-nine patients with malignant melanoma. *Cancer* (Phila.), 79: 611-619, 1966.

[59] McGovern VJ, Shaw HM, Milton GW, et al. Prognostic significance of the histological features of malignant melanoma. *Histopathology* (Oxf.), 3: 385-393, 1979.

[60] Amer MH, Al-Sarraf M, Vaitkevicius VK. Clinical presentation, natural history and prognostic factors in advanced malignant melanoma. *Surg. Gynecol. Obstet.* 1979; 149: 687-692.

[61] Khansur T, Sanders J, Das SK. Evaluation of staging workups in malignant melanoma. *Arch. Surg*. 1989, 124: 847-849.

[62] Iscoe N, Kersey P, Gapski J, et al: Predictive value of staging patients with clinical stage I malignant melanoma. *J. Plast. Reconstr. Surg*. 1987, 80: 233-239.

[63] Kirkwood JM, Myers JE, Vlock DR et al. Tomographic gallium- 67 citrate scanning: Useful new surveillance for metastatic melanoma. *Ann. Surg*. 1983; 198:102-107.

[64] Houghton AN, Meyers ML, Chapman PB. Medical treatment of metastatic melanoma. *Surgical Clinics of North America* 1996. Vol 76 (6), Pages 1343-1354.

[65] Quirt I, Verma S, Petrella T et al. Temozolomide for the treatment of metastatic melanoma. current oncology - volume 14, number 1.

[66] Rosenberg SA, Yang JC, Topalian SL, et al. Treatment of 283 consecutive patients with metastatic melanoma or renal cell cancer using high-dose bolus interleukin-2. *JAMA.* 1994, 271: 907-913.

[67] Ma D, Ariyan S. The use of isolated limb perfusion to manage recurrent malignant melanoma. *Clin. Plast. Surg*. 2000, 27: 441-450.

[68] Jafarian F, Powell J, Kokta V, Champagne M, Hatami A, McCuaig C, Marcoux D, Savard P.: Malignant melanoma in childhood and adolescence: report of 13 cases. *J. Am. Acad. Dermatol.* 2005 Nov;53(5):816-22

[69] Schmid-Wendtner MH, Berking C, Baumert J, Schmidt M, Sander CA, Plewig G, Volkenandt M.: Cutaneous melanoma in childhood and adolescence: an analysis of 36 patients. *J. Am. Acad. Dermatol.* 2002 Jun;46(6):874-9.

[70] Odom RB, James WD, Berger TG. Melanocytic nevi and neoplasms. In: James WD, Berger TG, Elston D (eds): Andrews' Diseases of the Skin. 9th ed. Philadelphia: WB Saunders, 2000, pp 881-889.

In: Metastatic Melanoma
Editors: S.A. Klein and J.P. Beckler
ISBN 978-1-61209-915-6

Chapter IV

The Role of Sentinel Lymph Node Biopsy in Patients with Thick (Breslow≥4mm) Cutaneous Melanoma

Justin Kelly** and M. J. Kerin
Dept of Academic Surgery, UCHG /NUIG,
Galway, Ireland

Abstract

An international panel, comprising a cross section of expert melanoma surgeons who have contributed data and leadership to further investigate the role of sentinel node biopsy (SNB) in melanoma, recently produced a consensus statement, outlining their overall interpretation of current evidence, as a guide to clinical treatment of patients with clinically localized melanoma. They agreed that SNB is standard of care in current practice because it is incorporated in staging guidelines from the AJCC, incorporated in the treatment guidelines from the National Comprehensive Cancer Network, and practiced by most specialty surgeons who treat melanoma in the United States, Australia and Western

* Email: justinjoshkelly@gmail.com, Phone: +35391495719.

Europe. The proven benefits for performing sentinel lymph node biopsy at the time of oncological wide local excision of a primary cutaneous melanoma in any patient, include both prognostic and staging information, the potential therapeutic impact of a completion lymph node dissection in those with a positive node and also has implications of nodal status for adjuvant therapy decisions or entry into pertinent clinical trials.

The prognosis for patients with a thick cutaneous melanoma (Breslow thickness >4 mm) is poor, with a 10-year melanoma specific mortality rate >50% and 5-year disease-free survival of <50%, causing both treatment difficulty and uncertainty for doctors, as well as patients. Because of this poor prognosis and high degree of synchronous metastatic disease at initial presentation in patients with a thick primary melanoma, the approach to the regional lymph nodes remains extremely controversial. The high risk of synchronous distant metastases is suggested by some to outweigh any benefit of staging or the possible therapeutic benefit of elective lymph node dissection in this group of patients. However, a significant amount of these patients survive without recurrent disease. Detection of lymph node involvement in thick melanomas may help to identify this group, particularly given that other factors (ulceration and Clark's level) seem to have less prognostic value in this group.

The aims of this book chapter are (1) to examine the possible prognostic and therapeutic role of sentinel lymph node biopsy as a potential standard of care for thick melanoma, (2) to evaluate the results of pertinent clinical trials and whether they can be extrapolated to thick melanomas and (3) to critically assess other emerging strategies targeting this difficult patient population.

Introduction

The key to survival for patients with melanoma is early detection and treatment of micro-metastatic disease as this may improve disease-free and overall survival rates [1]. The status of the regional lymph node basin has been widely shown to be the most important prognostic indicator for patients diagnosed with cutaneous melanoma. Melanomas less than 1mm rarely metastasise while at least 25% of melanomas between 1.5 and 4.0mm and greater than 60% of melanomas greater than 4.0mm thick will have lymph node metastases at presentation [2]. The outcome from melanoma also depends heavily on the stage at presentation. Patients with early stage disease (i.e. < 1mm thick) achieve long-term survival in more than 90% of cases.

However, for patients with melanomas greater than 1.0mm thickness the data is uninspiring with survival rates ranging from 50%-90% [2].

The introduction of the sentinel lymph node biopsy (SLNB) technique for the evaluation of patients with truncal and extremity melanoma by Morton et al in 1992 showed that the status of the SLN accurately represented the status of the entire nodal basin from which it was obtained. This study highlighted a novel technique of identifying patients with occult nodal metastasis who warranted possible further therapeutic lymphadenectomy and adjuvant therapy, whilst also sparing the remaining 80% of patients without regional disease the morbidity associated with a formal lymphadenectomy procedure [3].

The proven benefits for performing SLNB at the time of oncological wide local excision of a primary melanoma in any patient, include both prognostic and staging information, the potential therapeutic impact of a completion lymph node dissection in those with a positive SLN and also has implications of SLN status for adjuvant therapy decisions or entry into pertinent clinical trials.

A multivariate analysis involving 4750 patients with melanoma without clinical evidence of nodal metastases who underwent nodal staging by sentinel lymph node biopsy or elective nodal dissection confirmed that nodal status was the most significant predictor of disease-free survival [2]. Because the tumour status of the regional lymph nodes is the most single important prognostic factor for patients with melanoma, obtaining this information is essential in the management of these patients [4].

Conversely, clinicians opposed to the use of the sentinel node will argue that despite its prognostic importance, there is still no clear evidence to support a direct survival advantage from the procedure alone and that no effective adjuvant therapy has been discovered for these patients with lymph node metastatic disease [5, 6]. Confusion remains whether early completion lymphadenectomy imparts a survival advantage when compared directly to those patients who wait until clinically occult nodal metastatic disease becomes apparent. Numerous trials investigating the potential use of myriad adjuvant therapies including vaccines, differing combinations of chemotherapeutic agents, immunostimulants, cytokines and growth factors have failed to show any efficacy in trails to date [7-9].

The Evidence and Controversy Thus Far

The preliminary findings of the MSLT-1 trial (Multicentre Selective Lymphadenectomy Trial) represent the first randomised prospective clinical study to show a potential survival advantage to performing sentinel lymph node biopsy in patients with melanoma [10]. However, this study was limited to lesions between 1-4 mm in thickness. Thus, no firm data exists about the application of this proven staging method to patients with melanomatous lesions ≥4 mm in thickness. Indeed none of the other prospective trials in melanoma included patients with thick melanoma. Specifically in MSLT-1, for patients with intermediate thickness (1.2-3.5mm) primary melanomas, there was no significant difference in overall melanoma-related survival but the study did show improved disease-free survival in those patients who underwent the SLNB compared to those in the nodal observation arm group; thus there was a 26% reduction in the relative risk of recurrence (hazard ration 0.74; 95% confidence interval 0.59-0.93; P=0.009) which was durable for at least 10 years [10].

Furthermore, an international panel, comprising a cross section of expert melanoma surgeons who have contributed data and leadership to further investigate the role of SLNB in melanoma, recently produced a consensus statement, outlining their overall interpretation of current evidence, as a guide to clinical treatment of patients with clinically localized melanoma. They agreed that SLNB is standard of care in current practice because it is incorporated in staging guidelines from the AJCC, incorporated in the treatment guidelines from the National Comprehensive Cancer Network, and practiced by most specialty surgeons who treat melanoma in the United States, Australia and Western Europe [11].

There has been some international criticism leveled directly at the manner in which MSLT-1 was carried out and the conclusions derived from it [12, 13]. Stated evidence that, tiny sentinel nodal deposits of melanoma have no prognostic relevance and will not progress or disseminate further as determined by the hosts' immune system, is now accruing. Associating a poorer prognosis to these deposits is called prognostic false positivity; which can lead to patients being incorrectly upstaged, undergoing unnecessary completion lymphadenectomy and possibly unnecessary adjuvant therapy [14]. The results of the fourth interim analysis of MSLT-I support the hypothesis that prognostic false-positivity is the explanation for the large survival advantage claimed for patients having early lymphadenectomy versus delayed lymphadenectomy. Further detailed analysis of the results of MSLT-1 suggested that the incidence of prognostic false positivity is about 24% in patients with intermediate thickness melanoma and 34% for all patients [15]. Further credence is given to this stance from studies confirming that patients with these tiny deposits of nodal melanoma (ie detected by immunohistochemistry alone or <0.1mm in size), have similar prognosis to those who are sentinel node negative [16, 17].

The prognosis of patients with a thick melanoma (Breslow thickness ≥4 mm) is poor, with a 10-year melanoma specific mortality rate >50% [2] and 5-year disease-free survival of <50% [18], causing both treatment difficulty and uncertainty for doctors, as well as patients. Because of this high degree of synchronous metastatic disease at initial presentation and further systemic disease in patients who present with a thick primary melanoma [19], the approach to the regional lymph nodes remains extremely controversial [20, 21]. Because of the high risk that synchronous distant metastasis through vascular spread has already occurred in the majority of patients with a thick melanoma, there is widespread belief that control of the regional lymphatic basins, either for surgical cure or staging purposes, has potentially no bearing on final outcome [20-23]. However, a significant amount of these patients survive without recurrent disease. Detection of lymph node involvement in patients with thick melanomas may help to identify this group, particularly given that other factors (ulceration and Clark's level) seem to have less prognostic value in this subset of melanoma patients [22, 24]. Other experts believe that the poor prognosis and relatively high risk of regional metastatic disease in patients with thick non-ulcerated melanoma, without obvious regional or visceral metastatic disease, is not as large as previously thought [20-22, 24, 25] .

Some authors site compelling evidence that the assessment of the sentinel node in melanoma is of no benefit whatsoever, does not alter the course of melanoma that has metastasised and should be immediately abandoned from current practice [26].

Specific Problems with Sentinel Node Identification

There is growing concern surrounding the reliability of the SLN to accurately predict the disease status of the entire nodal basin. Specific problems have been identified in the head and neck region where the complexity and variablility of the interlacing network of cervical lymphatics was highlighted by O'Brien et al who showed a 34% discordance rate between the clinical prediction of lymphatic drainage and lymphoscintigraphy findings in 97 cases of cutaneous melanoma of the head and neck [27].

In experienced hands, the sentinel node can be identified in nearly 100% of cases, with a false-negative rate of < 5%. It can be performed in an outpatient setting and has little associated morbidity [28-31]. Conversely, the morbidity associated with lymph node dissection is substantial, with postoperative complications occurring in up to 39% of patients [32, 33], the majority of which are short-term ones including seroma, haematoma and abscess formation.

Regional nodal failures in all melanoma patients following a negative SLNB are uncommon and some studies have previously suggested that this was most commonly because conventional histological evaluation was unable to identify occult metastatic disease [34].

Various reasons have been suggested as to why SLNM fails. These include (1) when the primary lesion is overlying the draining lymph node basin, (2) learning curve of the performing surgeon / pathologist / nuclear medicine staff, (3) inappropriately high radioactivity level, (4) movement of the dye into the second or non-sentinel lymph node and (5) incorrect injection technique of the dye.

Patients undergoing SLNM for cutaneous melanoma should be managed via a multi-disciplinary team and the overall success rate of the procedure may be attributable in some part to this. It has been suggested that at least a 30 person learning curve be recommended for a surgeon performing these cases [28]. Experienced nuclear medicine staff is imperative as inappropriate administration of the radiolabelled isotope can directly affect the outcome of the procedure. Interpretation by a pathologist experienced in the technique of SLNB is also mandatory as a more thorough and detailed analysis of the SLNs is required than when examining a formal lymphadenectomy sample [30].

International Data for Thick Melanoma

A review of data currently available in the literature concerning other institutions' experience with SLNB in thick cutaneous melanoma is presented in Table 1. Concerning the prognostic role for SLNB in patients with thick cutaneous primary melanoma, the overall message from these studies remains unclear.

Gershenwald found in a retrospective study of 126 patients that, even though both the presence of ulceration and SLN status were statistically significant independent prognostic factors with respect to disease-free and overall survival, SLN status was the most powerful predictor of overall survival by univariate and multivariate analyses [22]. A negative SLNB was associated with a 35% increase in 3-year overall survival.

Table 1. (SLN: sentinel lymph node; +: positive; -: negative; DFS: disease free survival and OS: overall survival)

Study	*Gershenwald [22]*	*Essner [20]*	*Thompson [21]*	*Ferrone [35]*	*Carlson [36]*	*Gutzmer [38]*	*Gajdos [37]*
Year	2000	2002	2002	2002	2003	2008	2009
No of patients	126	113	172	126	114	152	228
Median age (years)	57	54	61	60	57	65	58
Median follow-up (months)	36	31	24	16	34	33	43
Mean tumour thickness (mm)	5.0	5.9	5.0 (median)	5.5	6.3	5.2	6.6
% ulceration present	50%	45%	53%	43%	35%	58%	34%
% of + SLN	39%	35%	30%	30%	32.5%	48%	47%
5 year DFS - + SLN - - SLN	48% 64%	34% 47%	29% 68%	32% 56%	3 years 31% 71%	26% 58%	—
5 year OS - + SLN - - SLN	54% 87%	50% 60%	41% 74%	—	57% 82%	37% 67%	47% 80%

Essner also found that the status of the SLN is predictive of 5 year disease free survival but not overall survival. This group also found no difference between ulcerated and non-ulcerated lesions in terms of survival [20].

Ferrone developed an interesting multivariate prognostic model for patients with thick cutaneous melanoma and found that the factors independently predictive of recurrence were age >60 years, depth >5.5 mm, ulceration, and SLN positivity, with the latter factor being the most significant prognosticator. The relative risk for an individual recurrence ranged from 1 in patients for whom no adverse factors were present to 29.4 when all factors were present. They concluded that these patients are prognostically heterogeneous, and all independently predictive factors should be considered when assessing an individual patient's risk of recurrence [35]. These findings associating a poorer outcome with SLN positivity and ulceration have been mirrored in several other studies [36-38].

Other Emerging Strategies

In an ideal oncological world, intra-operative evaluation of the sentinel node for metastatic disease would be ideal. This would allow a simultaneous completion lymphadenectomy occur if a positive deposit is immediately identified, preventing the costs and additional morbidity associated with a second operation. However, this would not be practical on a number of levels.

Frozen section analysis was studied in 368 patients with primary cutaneous melanoma ≥1mm or Carks level IV. 20% (74/368) of sentinel nodes were identified by traditional HandE and immunohistochemical stains, and further frozen sectioning only identified the metastases in 59% (44/74) of these patients [39]. This low sensitivity was confirmed in other subsequent studies [40, 41]. Frozen sectioning is also a technically difficult procedure to perform and often results in freezing artefact of the lymph node, rendering it unsuitable for further histological scrutiny.

Another recent development in the intra-operative identification of the sentinel node is called imprint cytology, which involves bisecting the node, imprinting and subsequently staining the relevant sections. One study involving 93 patients showed that imprint cytology had a sensitivity and specificity of 38% and 100% respectively (similar figure to that of frozen section) [42]. Even though it is easier to perform this procedure and without subsequent damage to the lymph node, the low sensitivity severely limits its use in the routine evaluation of the sentinel node.

Other algorithms of histological factors concerning the primary tumour have also been developed. These are able to stratify patients into high and minimal risk for sentinel node disease based on the analysis of their primary lesion, and upon validation, these models could possibly remove the use of the sentinel node procedure in those with minimal risk [43, 44].

Some molecular biology techniques for the staging of regional lymph nodes have yielded promising results [45]. Wang et al, using real-time PCR to identify tyrosine messenger RNA for the detection of micrometastatic lymph node disease, showed that this was a highly sensitive and clinically applicable method to detect micrometastases (tyrosine messenger RNA is found almost exclusively in melanocytes).

Furthermore, studies using reverse transcription and polymerase chain reaction to determine tyrosinase mRNA in peripheral blood, (which indicates the presence of circulating melanoma cells), showed that this may be a promising serum marker for melanoma staging and for predicting recurrence, prognosis and response to immune therapy [46]. The same group found that the amount of circulating tumour cells correlates with the tumour burden and that in patients with regression of melanoma metastases after immunotherapy, a decrease of the amount of tumour cells in the peripheral blood was observed [47], associating the rate of positivity with stage of the disease.

There is accumulating evidence to support the use of targeted ultrasound assessment of the regional nodal basin at the time of diagnosis of the primary tumour. It can now identify deposits as small as 3-4mm [48].

Voit et al showed that preoperative ultrasound and fine needle aspiration cytology can identify 65% of sentinel node metastases and thus reduce the need for surgical procedures on the sentinel node, allowing those patients identified to proceed directly to completion lymphadenectomy [49].

Conclusions

The management of a patient with a thick primary cutaneous melanoma remains somewhat unclear. It was previously thought that the assessment of their sentinel node was paramount, however others have long argued that given the relatively high degree of synchronous metastatic disease and further systemic disease at initial presentation, that surgical control of the regional nodal basins draining the primary melanoma is of no benefit. Unfortunately, this cohort of patients was not included in prospective trials comparing sentinel node biopsy/regional lymphadenectomy with nodal observation. Historically, some were offered adjuvant agents that were reputed to be efficacious in clinical trials. Apart from high dose interferon (which is both costly and has a number of common side-effects), none of the agents tried have any documented proven benefits as adjuvant therapy for melanoma, in terms of disease free and overall survival.

For those patients with intermediate thickness melanoma, the assessment of the sentinel node is strongly supported and recommended, however the extrapolation of this technique to thick melanoma remains controversial.

The evidence supports its use as a pertinent prognostic tool, as numerous studies have clearly shown that the status of the sentinel node (for thick melanoma) is the most important prognostic factor in terms of overall survival.

The obvious benefits include both prognostic and staging information, the potential therapeutic impact of a completion lymph node dissection in those with a positive sentinel node and the implications for adjuvant therapy decisions or entry into pertinent clinical trials. It is also important in providing patients with a better understanding of their prognosis. We should not definitively declare something as standard of care until we are convinced by credible results of appropriately designed studies published in peer reviewed journals [50].

Going forward, there is hope that newer adjuvant therapies will be discovered and developed that are more efficacious than those previously studied. Detailed histopathological assessment of the regional nodal basin will remain crucial such that adjuvant therapy may be more selective and thus more successful.

References

[1] Pacifico, M.D., R. Grover, and R. Sanders, Use of an early-detection strategy to improve disease control in melanoma patients. *Br. J. Plast. Surg.*, 2004. 57(2): p. 105-11.

[2] Balch, C.M., et al., Prognostic factors analysis of 17,600 melanoma patients: validation of the American Joint Committee on Cancer melanoma staging system. *J. Clin. Oncol.,* 2001. 19(16): p. 3622-34.

[3] Morton, D.L., et al., Technical details of intraoperative lymphatic mapping for early stage melanoma. *Arch. Surg.*, 1992. 127(4): p. 392-9.

[4] Shaw, H.M., et al., Prognostic histopathological factors in malignant melanoma. *Pathology,* 1985. 17(2): p. 271-4.

[5] Otley, C.C. and J.A. Zitelli, Review of sentinel lymph node biopsy and systemic interferon for melanoma: promising but investigational modalities. *Dermatol. Surg.,* 2000. 26(3): p. 177-80.

[6] Thomas, J.M. and E.J. Patocskai, The argument against sentinel node biopsy for malignant melanoma. *BMJ,* 2000. 321(7252): p. 3-4.

[7] Eggermont, A.M. and M. Gore, Randomized adjuvant therapy trials in melanoma: surgical and systemic. *Semin. Oncol.*, 2007. 34(6): p. 509-15.

[8] Sabel, M.S. and V.K. Sondak, Tumor vaccines: a role in preventing recurrence in melanoma? *Am. J. Clin. Dermatol.*, 2002. 3(9): p. 609-16.

[9] Spitler, L.E., Adjuvant therapy of melanoma. *Oncology* (Williston Park), 2002. 16(1 Suppl 1): p. 40-8.

[10] Morton, D.L., et al., Sentinel-node biopsy or nodal observation in melanoma. *N. Engl. J. Med.,* 2006. 355(13): p. 1307-17.

[11] Balch, C.M., et al., Sentinel node biopsy and standard of care for melanoma. *J. Am. Acad. Dermatol.*, 2009. 60(5): p. 872-5.

[12] Thomas, J.M., The place of sentinel node biopsy in melanoma after the Multicenter Selective Lymphadenectomy Trial. *ANZ J. Surg.*, 2006. 76(3): p. 98-9.

[13] Thomas, J.M., Concerns relating to the conduct and statistical analysis of the Multicenter Selective Lymphadenectomy Trial (MSLT-1) in patients with melanoma. *J. Plast. Reconstr. Aesthet. Surg.,* 2009. 62(4): p. 442-6.

[14] Thomas, J.M., Sentinel lymph node biopsy in malignant melanoma. *BMJ,* 2008. 336(7650): p. 902-3.

[15] Thomas, J.M., Prognostic false-positivity of the sentinel node in melanoma. *Nat. Clin. Pract. Oncol.*, 2008. 5(1): p. 18-23.

[16] Spanknebel, K., et al., Characterization of micrometastatic disease in melanoma sentinel lymph nodes by enhanced pathology: recommendations for standardizing pathologic analysis. *Am. J. Surg. Pathol.*, 2005. 29(3): p. 305-17.

[17] van Akkooi, A.C., et al., Clinical relevance of melanoma micrometastases (<0.1 mm) in sentinel nodes: are these nodes to be considered negative? *Ann. Oncol.*, 2006. 17(10): p. 1578-85.

[18] Salti, G.I., et al., Clinical node-negative thick melanoma. *Arch. Surg.*, 2002. 137(3): p. 291-5.

[19] Reintgen, D., et al., Recent advances in the care of the patient with malignant melanoma. *Ann. Surg.*, 1997. 225(1): p. 1-14.

[20] Essner, R., et al., Prognostic implications of thick (>or=4-mm) melanoma in the era of intraoperative lymphatic mapping and sentinel lymphadenectomy. *Ann. Surg. Oncol.,* 2002. 9(8): p. 754-61.

[21] Thompson, J.F. and H.M. Shaw, The prognosis of patients with thick primary melanomas: is regional lymph node status relevant, and does removing positive regional nodes influence outcome? *Ann. Surg. Oncol.*, 2002. 9(8): p. 719-22.

[22] Gershenwald, J.E., et al., Role for lymphatic mapping and sentinel lymph node biopsy in patients with thick (> or = 4 mm) primary melanoma. *Ann. Surg. Oncol.*, 2000. 7(2): p. 160-5.

[23] Crowley, N.J. and H.F. Seigler, The role of elective lymph node dissection in the management of patients with thick cutaneous melanoma. *Cancer,* 1990. 66(12): p. 2522-7.

[24] Cherpelis, B.S., et al., Sentinel lymph node micrometastasis and other histologic factors that predict outcome in patients with thicker melanomas. *J. Am. Acad. Dermatol.*, 2001. 44(5): p. 762-6.

[25] Kim, S.H., et al., Prognosis of thick cutaneous melanoma. *J. Am. Coll Surg.,* 1999. 188(3): p. 241-7.

[26] Medalie, N. and A.B. Ackerman, Sentinel node biopsy has no benefit for patients whose primary cutaneous melanoma has metastasized to a lymph node and therefore should be abandoned now. *Br. J. Dermatol.*, 2004. 151(2): p. 298-307.

[27] O'Brien, C.J., et al., Prediction of potential metastatic sites in cutaneous head and neck melanoma using lymphoscintigraphy. *Am. J. Surg.*, 1995. 170(5): p. 461-6.

[28] Morton, D.L., et al., Validation of the accuracy of intraoperative lymphatic mapping and sentinel lymphadenectomy for early-stage melanoma: a multicenter trial. Multicenter Selective Lymphadenectomy Trial Group. *Ann. Surg.*, 1999. 230(4): p. 453-63; discussion 463-5.

[29] Wrightson, W.R., et al., Complications associated with sentinel lymph node biopsy for melanoma. *Ann. Surg. Oncol.*, 2003. 10(6): p. 676-80.

[30] Cascinelli, N., et al., Sentinel lymph node biopsy in cutaneous melanoma: the WHO Melanoma Program experience. *Ann. Surg. Oncol.*, 2000. 7(6): p. 469-74.

[31] Jansen, L., et al., Reliability of sentinel lymph node biopsy for staging melanoma. *Br. J. Surg.*, 2000. 87(4): p. 484-9.

[32] Ingvar, C., C. Erichsen, and P.E. Jonsson, Morbidity following prophylactic and therapeutic lymph node dissection for melanoma--a comparison. *Tumori*, 1984. 70(6): p. 529-33.

[33] Sim, F.H., et al., Lymphadenectomy in the management of stage I malignant melanoma: a prospective randomized study. *Mayo Clin Proc*, 1986. 61(9): p. 697-705.

[34] Gershenwald, J.E., et al., Patterns of recurrence following a negative sentinel lymph node biopsy in 243 patients with stage I or II melanoma. *J. Clin. Oncol.*, 1998. 16(6): p. 2253-60.

[35] Ferrone, C.R., et al., Multivariate prognostic model for patients with thick cutaneous melanoma: importance of sentinel lymph node status. *Ann. Surg. Oncol.*, 2002. 9(7): p. 637-45.

[36] Carlson, G.W., et al., Sentinel lymph node mapping for thick (>or=4-mm) melanoma: should we be doing it? *Ann. Surg. Oncol.*, 2003. 10(4): p. 408-15.

[37] Gajdos, C., et al., Is there a benefit to sentinel lymph node biopsy in patients with T4 melanoma? *Cancer*, 2009. 115(24): p. 5752-60.

[38] Gutzmer, R., et al., Sentinel lymph node status is the most important prognostic factor for thick (> or = 4 mm) melanomas. *J. Dtsch Dermatol. Ges.*, 2008. 6(3): p. 198-203.

[39] Stojadinovic, A., et al., Value of frozen-section analysis of sentinel lymph nodes for primary cutaneous malignant melanoma. *Ann. Surg.*, 2002. 235(1): p. 92-8.

[40] Koopal, S.A., et al., Frozen section analysis of sentinel lymph nodes in melanoma patients. *Cancer,* 2000. 89(8): p. 1720-5.

[41] Tanis, P.J., et al., Frozen section investigation of the sentinel node in malignant melanoma and breast cancer. *Ann. Surg. Oncol.*, 2001. 8(3): p. 222-6.

[42] Creager, A.J., et al., Intraoperative evaluation of sentinel lymph nodes for metastatic melanoma by imprint cytology. *Cancer*, 2002. 94(11): p. 3016-22.

[43] Kruper, L.L., et al., Predicting sentinel node status in AJCC stage I/II primary cutaneous melanoma. *Cancer,* 2006. 107(10): p. 2436-45.

[44] Soong, S.J., et al., Predicting survival outcome of localized melanoma: an electronic prediction tool based on the AJCC Melanoma Database. *Ann. Surg. Oncol.* 17(8): p. 2006-14.

[45] Wang, X., et al., Detection of submicroscopic lymph node metastases with polymerase chain reaction in patients with malignant melanoma. *Ann. Surg.*, 1994. 220(6): p. 768-74.

[46] Brossart, P., et al., Hematogenous spread of malignant melanoma cells in different stages of disease. *J. Invest. Dermatol.*, 1993. 101(6): p. 887-9.

[47] Brossart, P., et al., A polymerase chain reaction-based semiquantitative assessment of malignant melanoma cells in peripheral blood. *Cancer Res.*, 1995. 55(18): p. 4065-8.

[48] Bafounta, M.L., et al., Ultrasonography or palpation for detection of melanoma nodal invasion: a meta-analysis. *Lancet Oncol.*, 2004. 5(11): p. 673-80.

[49] Voit, C., et al., Ultrasound morphology criteria predict metastatic disease of the sentinel nodes in patients with melanoma. *J. Clin. Oncol.* 28(5): p. 847-52.

[50] Connelly, T.J., Lymphatic mapping and sentinel lymph node biopsy. *J. Am. Acad. Dermatol.*, 2002. 46(4): p. 640; author reply 640.

Reviewed by:

Prof H P Redmond,
Professor and Chair of the Department of Surgery,
University College Cork,
Cork University Hospital,
Wilton,
Cork City,
Ireland.
Email: mary.ahern@ucc.ie, henry.redmond@mailp.hse.ie
Phone: +353 214922371

In: Metastatic Melanoma
Editors: S.A. Klein and J.P. Beckler
ISBN 978-1-61209-915-6

Chapter V

Hormone Replacement Therapy and Malignant Melanoma

Marcia S. Driscoll[1]* and Jane M. Grant-Kels[2]
[1]Clinical Associate Professor, Department of Dermatology
University of Maryland School of Medicine
419 W. Redwood Street, Suite 160
Baltimore, Maryland 21201, USA
[2]Professor and Chairman, Department of Dermatology
University of Connecticut Health Center
Dermatology Residency Director
Director of Dermatopathology and the
Cutaneous Oncology and Melanoma Program
21 South Road
Farmington, Connecticut 06030, USA

Abstract

Controversy concerning whether pregnancy portends a poor prognosis for women diagnosed with malignant melanoma (MM) has led to questions concerning the effect of *exogenous* hormones (hormone replacement therapy, oral contraceptive pills) on MM prognosis.

* Phone: 410-328-3167; Fax: 410-328-1323; E-mail: bdriscollent@msn.com.

Since the 1970's, many epidemiologic studies have attempted to address the impact of oral contraceptive pill (OCP) use and relative risk of MM. Far fewer studies have addressed the influence of hormone replacement therapy (HRT) on relative risk of MM or on prognosis in those diagnosed with MM. Herein we review the history of the controversial relationship between hormones and MM, and analyze the relevant studies. Overall the evidence to date does not suggest a link between exogenous hormones and a woman's risk of developing MM.

Introduction

The question of a hormonal influence on MM originated with multiple case reports dating back to the 1950's [1-5]. Pack and Scharnagel [1] reviewed over 1000 cases of MM, and of 10 patients who were diagnosed during pregnancy, 5 died within 30 months of diagnosis. Reports such as these suggested either a poor outcome for those diagnosed with MM during pregnancy, or transformation of nevi into MM under the influence of pregnancy-related hormones. The impact of homones was supported by the observation that the incidence of MM increases steadily during the reproductive years, then declines after menopause [6]. More recently, investigation into the relationship between estrogen receptor β (ERβ) and melanoma has proven interesting; ERβ's expression in both nevi and melanoma is significantly greater than that of estrogen receptor α (ERα) expression [7,8].

However, our recent extensive review of the literature [9] does not support a relationship between either endogenous homones (pregnancy) or exogenous hormones, i.e. OCPs or HRT. The clinical relevance of the presence of ERβ in MMs will only be determined through continued investigation. One small study reported by De Giorgi et al. [7] evaluated MMs from 12 patients with MM, and observed decreased ERβ expression in thicker MMs (> 1mm Breslow depth) compared to thin MMs (≤ 1 mm Breslow depth), suggesting that a loss ERβ expression may portend a worse prognosis, as has been observed in other types of malignancy [10]. In this chapter, we focus on the relationship between exogenous hormones and MM by reviewing 1) risk of MM due to OCP use, 2) risk of MM associated with HRT and OCP use, and 3) prognosis of MM associated with OCP and HRT use. Finally, we offer recommendations on counseling patients diagnosed with MM concerning future treatment with OCPs or HRT.

Risk of Melanoma Associated with OCP Use

The majority of evidence that is relevant to a discussion of whether HRT is linked to MM is derived from the studies addressing whether or not OCPs increase one's risk of MM. The largest number of studies address this specific question and date back to the 1970s. The majority of these studies are case-control studies, where risk is typically expressed as an estimate of relative risk (RR) or odds ratio (OR). For the specific studies in this section, RR is defined as the incidence of MM in those exposed to OCPs / incidence of MM in those never exposed to OCPs; OR is defined as the odds of MM occurring in those exposed to OCPs / odds of MM occurring in those not exposed to OCPs. In this chapter study results will be discussed including a calculated RR or OR, along with a 95% confidence interval (CI). If the RR or OR = 1, this signifies no difference between the groups; if the 95% CI includes 1, then it cannot be ruled out that the RR is 1, and therefore no difference between groups exists.

The majority of studies, primarily of case-control design, have not observed an enhanced risk of MM due to OCP use. A review of 22 studies [11-32] did not show an impact of "ever use" of OCPs compared with those who never used OCPs. Two of the earliest reports showed that OCPs increased a woman's risk of MM. These two studies published in 1977 and 1981 were based on a cohort of women enrolled in the California Kaiser-Permanente Health Plan [11,12]. Potential confounding factors include lack of measure for sun exposure or outdoor activity. Indeed, a sample analysis from the 1981 report suggested that OCP users were more likely to sunbathe than did non-OCP users who developed MM [12]. A few other studies suggested a slightly increased risk of MM associated with a long duration of OC use [15, 17, 18, 26]. These earlier studies have a number of potential flaws: small numbers of patients with MM, lack of control for potential confounders (especially sun exposure and skin type), or lack of statistical significance of their results.

The risk of MM in OCP users was analyzed in a large, prospective study in the Nurses' Health Study (NHS) and NHS II cohorts, and a significant increase in risk was observed in *current* users of OCPs compared to never users (combined RR = 2.0; 95% CI 1.2 - 3.4), but risk of MM was not increased in *past* OCP users, even with more than 10 years of OCP use (combined RR = 1.4; 95% CI 0.8 – 2.5) [13].

The strengths of the study include its large population and prospective design, but the disparity in results compared with the majority of other studies may be related to the small sample size of 23 MM cases in the *current* user group (those that showed increased risk of MM) compared to 165 cases of MM in the category of *past* users.

In addition, the investigators state that their study could be limited by "lack of information on sunbathing habits and the use of sunscreen and other protective measures during periods of OC use [13]."

Koomen and colleagues [14] reported the most recent case-control study of OCs and risk of MM in 2008. Similar to the NHS I and II study results, OCP use of at least 0.5 years was associated with a significantly increased risk of MM (OR 1.28, 95% CI 1.06 – 1.54). While this study included a large number of MM cases and controls (778 and 4072, respectively) the methodology differed from other studies. The investigators linked pathology and pharmacy databases from the Netherlands, so the study lacks data concerning important potential confounding factors, such as sun exposure, sunburn history, skin type, and eye and hair color [14].

The most convincing evidence for analysis of risk of MM due to OCP use arises from combining large numbers of case-control studies, since individual studies often included small numbers of patients. Such analyses include 2 recent meta-analyses, and a pooled analysis of 10 case-control studies.

These studies concur that OCPs do not appear to impact a woman's risk of MM [33-35]. A meta-analysis of 18 studies published between 1977– 1996 reported a summation OR of 0.95; 95% CI, 0.82-1.15 [33].

A second meta-analysis of 18 studies suggested no impact of OCPs on risk of MM [34]. The latter reported summary ORs, using both fixed effects and random effects models, of OR = 0.95; CI 0.87-1.04 and 0.87-1.05, respectively, using a total of 3796 cases and 9442 controls. A 2002 pooled analysis of 10 case-control studies, including 2391 cases and 3199 controls, reported no relationship between risk of MM and ever use of OCPs (pooled OR 0.86; 95% CI 0.74-1.01) [35]. Furthermore, there was no relationship between risk of MM and OC length of use, age at first use, or current use.

These investigators meticulously restricted their analysis to studies which accounted for important potential confounding factors, including family history of MM, skin type, and sun exposure. The latter pooled analysis [35], and our review of the literature to date, show that OCP use does not play a role in the development of MM.

Risk of MM Associated with HRT Use

Compared to the risk of MM related to OCPs, far fewer studies have examined the risk of MM and use of HRT. These are primarily case-control studies dating back to the 1970s, which do not show an increased risk of MM due to HRT. Of 12 investigations [11,14,17-19,21,23,30-32, 35,36], only 2 have shown an augmented risk of MM related to HRT use [17,36]. A 1994 study reported by Holly and colleagues [17] reported an enhanced risk of MM associated with use of HRT, primarily in those who received HRT after hysterectomy, but not after natural menopause.

In addition, those who received HRT for less than 5 years after bilateral oophorectomy, or received HRT for at least 2 years after one ovary was removed showed an enhanced risk of MM.

However, this study had small numbers of MM cases, did not account for all the known potential confounders, and the length of use of HRT was not associated with an increased risk, as might be expected if a causal relationship existed. Koomen et al. [14] reported an enhanced risk of MM associated with HRT use (OR = 2.08; 95% CI 1.37-3.14), but as discussed above in regard to OCPs, this study did not account for important potential confounding factors, including sun exposure, since their database linked pharmacy records to pathology records.

Effect of HRT and OCPs on Prognosis in Patients with MM

The best way to evaluate a possible effect of HRT or OCPs on prognosis after a diagnosis of MM is through a randomized controlled trial, evaluating women with MM who requested hormone therapy (HRT or OCPs) with randomization to either a hormone therapy or placebo group [37]. A large trial such as this has not been performed, and we can only rely on existing studies to draw conclusions.

MacKie et al. [37] conducted a prospective observational study which addresses the impact of HRT on MM prognosis, reported in 2004. They studied 206 women diagnosed with localized MM (American Joint Committee on Cancer Stage I and II), who were followed for a minimum of 5 years.

A general practitioner or gynecologist prescribed HRT to 83 women for a time period ranging from 1 month to 19 years, and compared them with 123 women who did not receive HRT at any time.

When multivariate regression analysis was performed with adjustment for ulceration, tumor thickness, and age, there was a significantly increased survival for woman treated with HRT ($p = 0.007$) compared to those who never received HRT. This study suggests that HRT does not adversely affect prognosis for women diagnosed with localized MM, and possibly exerts a beneficial effect on survival.

Counseling Patients with Melanoma Concerning Future Use of OCPs or HRT

As discussed previously in this chapter, there are few data that *directly* address the effect of OCPs or HRT on prognosis for women previously diagnosed with MM. Our review showed that neither OCPs nor HRT increase one's risk of developing MM.

As for HRT, a sole observational, prospective study [37] showed no adverse effect on survival when HRT was prescribed to women with localized MM. If we can extrapolate from *endogenous* hormone effects on MM prognosis, then 3 small studies of *pregnancy* after a diagnosis of MM likewise had no detrimental effect on survival [38-40]. Likewise, 6 case-control studies and 2 large population-based studies observed no effect of pregnancy on prognosis for women diagnosed with localized MM as discussed in detail in our previous review [9].

Therefore our recommendations on counseling women diagnosed with localized MM about future use of OCPs or HRT, is that hormonal therapy should not be withheld if no appropriate alternative therapy exists [41].

Advising a patient should of course be individualized, especially for the patient with a greater likelihood for recurrence of disease (primary tumor depth > 1mm, ulcerated MM, etc.) or advanced MM.

In these latter scenarios, one might consider deferring hormonal therapy for 2-3 years, which is the time period in which MM recurrence is most likely.

Conclusion

While early case reports suggested a negative impact of hormones on the prognosis of MM, more recent studies do not show an adverse effect of OCPs or HRT on MM. In addition, while investigations into ERβ receptors expressed in MMs and nevi are intriguing, their clinical relevance has yet to be determined. In this chapter, we reviewed studies concerning OCPs and HRT and the risk of MM, and a sole study concerning impact of HRT on prognosis for women diagnosed with localized MM. Neither OCPs nor HRT appear to increase a woman's risk or alter her prognosis for MM. Although not discussed in detail in this chapter, our previous literature reviews have demonstrated that pregnancy-related homones do not appear to influence a woman's risk of MM nor affect prognosis for those with localized MM, lending more support to our conclusion. In sum, there is little evidence for a link between hormonal therapy and MM at present.

We counsel women diagnosed with localized MM that future use of OCPs or HRT is not absolutely contraindicated if no acceptable alternative exists. In patients at higher risk for recurrence, it may be reasonable to avoid hormonal therapy for 2 to 3 years, as this is the interval during which MM recurrence is most likely. For the woman with advanced stages of melanoma, more caution should be exercised, and counseling performed on a case-by-case basis.

References

[1] Pack GT, Scharnagel IM. The prognosis for malignant melanoma in the pregnant woman. *Cancer* 1951;4:324-334.

[2] Byrd BF, McGanity WJ. The effect of pregnancy on the clinical course of malignant melanoma. *South Med. J.* 1954;47:196-200.

[3] Conybeare RC. Malignant melanoma in pregnancy: report of three cases. *Obstet. Gynecol.* 1964;24:451-454.

[4] Riberti C, Marola G, Bertani A. Malignant melanoma: the adverse effects of pregnancy. *Br. J. Plast. Surg.* 1981;34:338-339.

[5] Pennington DG. Multiple primary melanomas in pregnancy: a case report. *Br. J. Plast. Surg.* 1983;36:260-261.

[6] Strouse JJ, Fears TR, Tucker MA, et al. Pediatric melanoma: risk factor and survival analysis of the surveillance, epidemiology, and end results database. *J. Clin. Oncol.* 2005;23:4735-4741.

[7] de Giorgi V, Mavilia C, Massi D, et al. Estrogen receptor expression in cutaneous melanoma. *Arch. Dermatol.* 2009;145:30-36.

[8] de Giorgi V, Gori A, Grazzini M, et al. The initiation and progression of melanoma: estrogens or estrogen receptors? *Melanoma Res.* 2010;20:64-65.

[9] Driscoll MS, Grant-Kels JM. Hormones, nevi and melanoma: an approach to the patient. *J. Am. Acad. Dermatol.* 2007;57:919-931.

[10] Driscoll MS, Grant-Kels JM. Estrogen receptor expression in cutaneous melanoma. *Arch. Dermatol.* 2009;145:73-75.

[11] Beral V, Ramcharan S, Faris R. Malignant melanoma and oral contraceptive use among women in California. *Br. J. Cancer* 1977;36:804-809.

[12] Ramcharan S, Pellegrin FA, Ray R, et al. The Walnut Creek Contraceptive Drug Study, Vol III. Bethesda, MD, Center for Population Research, *National Institute of Health*, 1981.

[13] Feskanich D, Hunter DJ, Willett WC, et al. Oral contraceptive use and risk of melanoma in premenopausal women. *Br. J. Cancer* 1999;81: 918-923.

[14] Koomen ER, Joosse A, Herings RM, et al. Estrogens, oral contraceptives and hormonal replacement therapy increase the incidence of cutaneous melanoma: a population-based case-control study. *Ann. Oncol.* 2009;20:358-364.

[15] Adam SA, Sheaves SA, Wright NH, et al. A case-control study of the possible association between oral contraceptives and malignant melanoma. *Br. J. Cancer* 1981;44:45-50.

[16] Bain C, Hennekens Ch, Speizer FE, et al. Oral contraceptive use and malignant melanoma. *J. Natl. Cancer Inst.* 1982;68:537-539.

[17] Holly EA, Weiss NS, Liff JM. Cutaneous melanoma in relation to exogenous hormones and reproductive factors. *J. Natl. Cancer Inst.* 1983;70:827-831.

[18] Beral V, Evans S, Shaw H, et al. Oral contraceptive use and malignant melanoma in Australia. *Br. J. Cancer* 1984;50:681-685.

[19] Holman CDJ, Armstrong BK, Heenan PJ. Cutaneous malignant melanoma in women: exogenous sex hormones and reproductive factors. *Br. J. Cancer* 1984; 50:673-80.

[20] Helmrich SP, Rosenberg L, Kaufman DW, et al. Lack of an elevated risk of malignant melanoma in relation to oral contraceptive use. *J. Natl. Cancer Inst.* 1984;72:617-20.

[21] Gallagher RP, Elwood JM, Hill GB, et al. Reproductive factors, oral contraceptives and risk of malignant melanoma: Western Canada melanoma study. *Br. J. Cancer*. 1985; 52:901-907.

[22] Green A, Bain C. Hormonal factors and melanoma in women. *Med. J. Aust*. 1985; 142:446-448.

[23] Osterlind A, Tucker MA, Stone BJ, et al. The Danish case-control study of cutaneous malignant melanoma. III. Hormonal and reproductive factors in women. *Int. J. Cancer* 1988;42:821-4.

[24] Zanetti R, Franceschi S, Rosso S, et al. Cutaneous malignant melanoma in females: the role of hormonal and reproductive factors. *Int. J. Epidemiol.* 1990;19:522-526.

[25] Hannaford PC, Villard-Mackintosh L, Vessey MP, et al. Oral contraceptives and malignant melanoma. *Br. J. Cancer* 1991;63:430-433.

[26] Lê MG, Cabanes PA, Desvignes V, et al. Oral contraceptive use and risk of cutaneous malignant melanoma in a case-control study of French women. *Cancer Causes Control* 1992; 3:199-205.

[27] Palmer JR, Rosenberg L, Strom BL, et al. Oral contraceptive use and risk of cutaneous malignant melanoma. *Cancer Causes Control* 1992;3:547-554.

[28] Holly EA, Cress RD, Ahn DK. Cutaneous melanoma in women. III. Reproductive factors and oral contraceptive use. *Am. J. Epidemiol.* 1995;141:943-50.

[29] Westerdahl J, Olsson H, Masback A, et al. Risk of malignant melanoma in relation to drug intake, alcohol, smoking and hormonal factors. *Br. J. Cancer* 1996; 73:1126-31.

[30] Smith MA, Fine JA, Barnhill RL, et al. Hormonal and reproductive influences and risk of melanoma in women. *Int. J. Epidemiol.* 1998 Oct; 27:751-7.

[31] Lea CS, Holly EA, Hartge P, et al. Reproductive risk factors for cutaneous melanoma in women: a case-control study. *Am. J. Epidemiol.* 2007;165:505-513.

[32] Naldi L, Altieri A, Imberti GL, et al. Cutaneous malignant melanoma in women. Phenotypic characteristics, sun exposure, and hormonal factors: a case-control study from Italy. *Ann. Epidmiol.* 2005;15:545-50.

[33] Gefeller O, Hassan K, Wille L. Cutaneous malignant melanoma in women and the role of oral contraceptives. *Br. J. Dermatol.* 1998; 38:122-124.

[34] Pfahlberg A, Hassan K, Wille L, et al. Systematic review of case-control studies: oral contraceptives show no effect on melanoma risk. *Public Health Rev* 1997;25: 309-15.

[35] Karagas MR, Stuckel TA, Dykes J, et al. A pooled analysis of 10 case-control studies of melanoma and oral contraceptive use. *Br. J. Cancer* 2002;86:1085-1092

[36] Holly EA, Cress RD, Ahn DK. Cutaneous melanoma in women: ovulatory life, menopause, and use of exogenous estrogens. *Cancer Epidemiol. Biomarkers Prev.* 1994;3:661-668.

[37] MacKie RM, Bray CA. Hormone replacement therapy after surgery for stage 1 or 2 cutaneous melanoma. *Br. J. Cancer*. 2004;90:770-772.

[38] Reintgen DS, McCarty KS, Vollmer R, et al. Malignant melanoma and pregnancy. *Cancer* 1985;55:1340-1344.

[39] MacKie RM, Bufalino R, Morabito A, et al. Lack of effect of pregnancy on outcome of melanoma. *Lancet* 1991;337:653-655.

[40] Lens MB, Rosdahl I, Albom A, et al. Effect of pregnancy on survival in women with cutaneous malignant melanoma. *J. Clin. Oncol.* 2004; 22:4369-4375.

[41] Durvasula R, Ahmed SM, Vashisht A, et al. Hormone replacement therapy and malignant melanoma: to prescribe or not to prescribe? *Climacteric* 2002;5:197-200.

In: Metastatic Melanoma
Editors: S.A. Klein and J.P. Beckler
ISBN 978-1-61209-915-6

Chapter VI

Novel Diagnostic and Prognostic Biomarkers and Molecular Therapeutic Targets in Aggressive, Metastatic and Recurrent Melanomas

***Murielle Mimeault*[*] *and Surinder K. Batra*[‡]**
Department of Biochemistry and Molecular Biology, College of Medicine, University of Nebraska Medical Center, Omaha, Nebraska, USA

Abstract

Cutaneous melanomas are the malignant and aggressive tumors of skin with extremely poor survival rates for the patients diagnosed with locally invasive and metastatic disease stages. Despite intensive research has led in last few years to an improvement of the curative treatment of

[*] Department of Biochemistry and Molecular Biology, College of Medicine, University of Nebraska Medical Center, Omaha, Nebraska 68198-5870, U.S.A., Phone: (402)559-5455; Fax: (402)559-6650; Email: mmimeault@unmc.edu.

[‡] Department of Biochemistry and Molecular Biology, College of Medicine, University of Nebraska Medical Center, Omaha, Nebraska 68198-5870, U.S.A., Phone: (402)559-5455; Fax: (402)559-6650; Email: sbatra@unmc.edu.

early-stage cutaneous melanomas by tumor surgical resection, ionizing radiation, systemic chemotherapy, immunotherapy and/or adjuvant stem cell-based therapies, the locally advanced and disseminated melanomas are generally resistant to conventional therapies and result to the death of cancer patients. The rapid progression of primary melanomas to locally invasive and/or metastatic disease stages remains a major obstacle for an early effective diagnosis and a curative therapeutic intervention for melanoma patients. Importantly, recent advances in the melanoma research have led to the identification of different gene products that are frequently implicated in the malignant transformation of melanocytic cells into melanoma cells, including melanoma stem/progenitor cells, during cancer initiation and progression to locally advanced and metastatic disease stages. These oncogenic events include the occurrence of activating mutations in distinct oncogenes such as v-Raf murine sarcoma viral oncogene homolog B1 (*B-RAF*) or neuroblastoma RAS viral oncogene homolog (*N-Ras*). The enhanced expression and activities of diverse growth factor signaling elements such as epidermal growth factor receptor (EGFR), sonic hedgehog, Wnt/β-catenin, Notch and vascular endothelial growth factor (VEGF)/VEGF-R receptors in melanoma cells also represent common molecular events associated with melanoma progression, metastases at distant sites, treatment resistance and disease relapse. Of therapeutic relevance, these deregulated signaling transduction components constitute new potential biomarkers and therapeutic targets of great clinical interest for improving the efficacy of current diagnostic and prognostic methods and management of patients diagnosed with locally advanced, metastatic and/or relapsed melanomas.

Keywords: Cutaneous melanomas, Melanoma cells, Melanoma stem/ progenitor cells, Growth factors, Invasion, Angiogenesis, Metastases, Drug resistance, Diagnosis, Prognosis, Cancer therapy, Molecular targeting.

Abbreviations

ABC, ATP-binding cassette; EGFR, epidermal growth factor receptor; IL, interleukin; INF, interferon, KIT, stem cell factor receptor; HA, hyaluronan; MAPK, mitogen-activated protein kinase; MEK, extracellular signal-related kinase kinase; MIC-1, macrophage inhibitory cytokine-1; MMPs, matrix metalloproteinases; NF-κB, nuclear factor-kappaB; PI3K, phosphatidylinositol 3'-kinase; PTCH, hedgehog patched receptor; PTEN, phosphatase and tensin homolog deleted on chromosome 10; SHH, sonic hedgehog ligand; SMO, smoothened; VEGF, vascular endothelial growth factor; VEGFR-2, vascular endothelial growth factor receptor-2; Wnt, Wingless ligand.

Introduction

Cutaneous malignant melanomas are highly aggressive tumors that represent the major cause of mortality among skin cancers [1,2]. Although the localized cutaneous melanomas diagnosed in the early stages are usually curable by surgical resection of malignant tumors, the rapid progression to invasive and metastatic melanomas is generally associated with a poor median survival of 6 to 12 months and a five year survival rate of less than 10% [1-5]. The therapeutic options for the patients with unresectable melanomas and distant metastases such as lungs, liver, brain and other organs consisting to the radiation therapy and/or chemotherapy are only *palliative*, aiming to improve the *quality of life* of patients [5-7]. Especially, the standard treatment with alkylating agent, decarbazine (also termed DTCI) or its orally active analog temozolomide, which is the most largely used chemotherapeutic drug for treating patients with advanced melanoma, alone or in combination therapy with other cytotoxic drugs and/or adjuvant hormonal or immunotherapeutic compounds, is usually ineffective and culminate to the development of drug resistance and disease relapse [8-10].

Importantly, recent advances in melanoma research have led to the establishment of the molecular transforming events that may contribute to melanoma initiation and progression and treatment resistance of melanoma cells, including melanoma stem/progenitor cells with stem cell-like properties. Especially, it has been observed that the persistent activation of different oncogenic signaling cascades initiated in an autocrine or a paracrine manner by distinct growth factors and cytokines through their cognate receptors is typically involved in the sustained proliferation, survival, invasion and metastases at distant sites of melanoma cells and angiogenic process [2,11-20]. Among them, the up-regulated expression levels and/or activities of epidermal growth factor receptor (EGFR), sonic hedgehog, Wnt/β-catenin, stem cell factor (SCF) receptor KIT, Notch, rearranged during transfection (c-RET) receptor tyrosine kinase and vascular endothelial growth factor (VEGF)/VEGFR receptors frequently occur during melanoma etiopathogenesis and progression (Figure 1) [2,11-21]. These tumorigenic cascades can provide critical functions for the tumor growth, metastases at distant sites, treatment resistance and disease relapse [2,11-21]. In addition, the enhanced secretion of diverse inflammatory cytokines such as macrophage inhibitory cytokine-1 (MIC-1), interleukin-2 (IL-2), hypoxia-inducible factor-1 (HIF-1), basic fibroblast growth factor (bFGF) and VEGF by melanoma cells and/or tumor stromal cells also may cooperate to promote the progression of localized melanomas to invasive and metastatic disease stages [14,15,17,18,20,22,23]. In this matter, we review the most recent advancements on the establishment of molecular transforming events and deregulated gene products that are often implicated in melanoma initiation and progression to locally invasive and metastatic disease stages and which may be exploited to develop novel multiplex biomarker detection methods for the diagnosis and prognosis and multitargeted therapies for treating the melanoma patients.

Molecular Transforming Events Associated with the Pathogenesis of Cutaneous Malignant Melanomas

Several intrinsic and environmental factors may contribute to promote the development of cutaneous melanomas. Among the factors that may predispose for melanoma formation, there are a frequent sun exposure, intense oxidative stress and chronic inflammation as well as the accumulation of different oncogenic events during chronological aging that may cause severe DNA damages and genomic instability in the skin cells [1,2,14,16-18,24-29]. Moreover, an enhanced risk for an individual to develop cutaneous melanomas may be promoted by specific genetic alterations such as the activating mutations in the v-Raf murine sarcoma viral oncogene homolog B1 (*B-RAF* V600E) or neuroblastoma RAS viral oncogene homolog (*N-Ras*) [1,2,16,30-35].

On the other hand, other transforming events often associated with melanoma etiopathogenesis include the inactivation or down-regulation of diverse tumor suppressor genes such as phosphatase and tensin homolog deleted on chromosome 10 (PTEN), $p16^{INK4A}$, inhibitors of cyclin-dependent kinases $p21^{WAP1}$ and $p27^{KIP1}$, *p53* and/or retinoblastoma (*pRb*) as well as the overexpression of anti-apoptotic factors such as Bcl-2 [17,18,27,29,34,36-40]. Also, the telomere attrition combined with a sustained stimulation of diverse developmental signaling cascades initiated by distinct growth factors, chemokines and cytokines typically occur in melanoma cells and may contribute to their acquisition of a more malignant behavior and disease progression to locally invasive and metastatic stages (Figure 1) [1,2,10,11,14,16,17,24-28,36,37]. Among the growth factor cascades that are often deregulated in melanoma cells during disease progression, there are EGFR, sonic hedgehog, Wnt/β-catenin, Notch, KIT, Nodal/Cripto-1 and VEGF/VEGFR pathways [17,18,21].

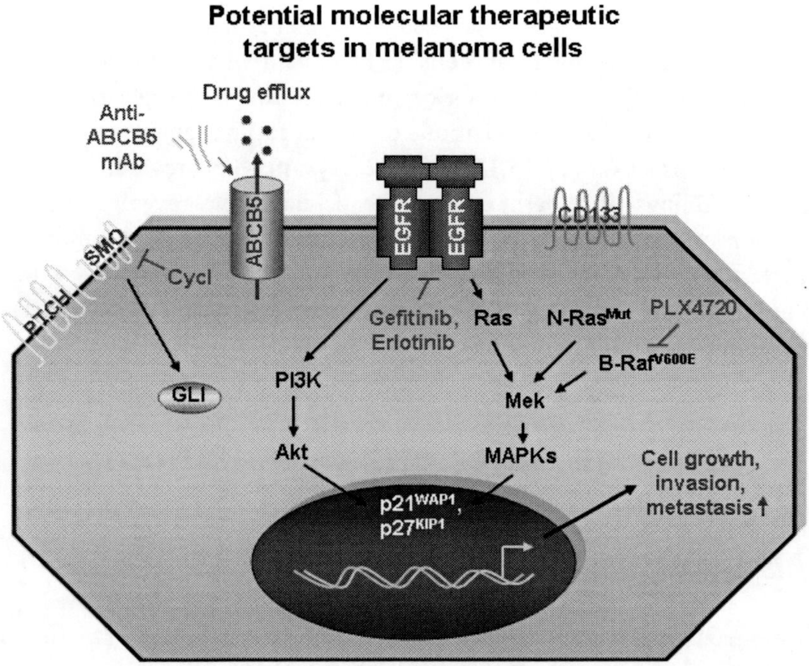

Figure 1. Novel targeted therapies against locally advanced, aggressive and metastatic melanomas. The scheme shows the intracellular signaling cascades induced through the activation of distinct growth factor pathways which may provide critical roles for the sustained growth, survival, migration, invasion, metastases and/or drug resistance of melanoma cells, including melanoma-initiating cells, through the up-regulation of the expression levels of different target gene products. The target gene products include cyclin D1, c-Myc, Bcl-2, Nodal, N-cadherin, matrix metalloproteinase (MMPs), urokinase-type plasminogen activator (uPA), cyclooxygenase (COX-2) and vascular epidermal growth factor (VEGF). The potential blockade of these tumorigenic signaling pathways by using a selective inhibitor of receptor tyrosine kinases (RTKs) such as EGFR (gefitinib or erlotinib), smoothened (SMO) hedgehog signaling element (cyclopamine "Cycl") and oncogenic B-Raf (E600V) mutant as well as a monoclonal antibody (mAb) directed against the stem cell-like markers, CD133 and ABCB5 multidrug transporter are also indicated.

These tumorigenic cascades may cooperate for the acquisition of more malignant phenotypes and survival advantages by melanoma stem/progenitor cells and their progenies, metastases at distant sites, treatment resistance and disease relapse.

In addition, the development of cutaneous melanomas is generally accompanied by the extensive changes in the local tumor microenvironment of melanoma cells, including in extracellular matrix (ECM) components and the stromal cells [14,15,17,18,20,22,23]. More particularly, the tumor-associated myofibroblasts or bone marrow-derived cells such as hematopoietic stem cells (HSCs), endothelial progenitor cells (EPCs) and mesenchymal stem cells (MSCs), can contribute in a paracrine manner through the release of diverse mitotic factors to their acquisition of a more malignant behavior and angiogenesis process [14,15,17,18,20,22,23]. In this regard, we review accumulating lines of experimental evidence that have revealed the critical implication of melanoma cells with stem cell-like properties in tumor growth and metastases at distant sites as well as the potential biomarkers that may be used as prognostic indicator of the disease progression and molecular targets for eradicating the total tumor mass of melanoma cells.

Critical Functions of Melanoma Stem/Progenitor Cells in Cutaneous Melanoma Formation and Progression

Cutaneous melanomas appear to arise from the malignant transformation of adult pluripotent epidermal neural crest stem cells (eNCSC) or their progenitors localized in the bulge areas at the basis of hair follicles into tumorigenic melanoma stem/progenitor cells [17,18,41-43]. In support with the critical functions of melanoma stem/progenitor cells, also designated melanoma- or metastasis-initiating cells, in the melanoma development and metastases at distant sites, the subpopulations of highly tumorigenic melanoma cells expressing the stem cell-like markers such as CD133, nestin, aldehyde dehydrogenase (ALDH), neural crest nerve gowth factor receptor (CD271) and/or high levels of ATP-binding cassette (ABC) multidrug resistance transporters such as multidrug resistance-1 (*MDR-1*) encoding P-glycoprotein (P-gp), ABCG2 and ABCB5 have been identified *in situ* and isolated from primary and secondary melanoma tumors, peripheral blood mononuclear cell (PBMC) population and/or established melanoma cell lines [17,18,41,44-54].

It has been shown that these immature melanoma stem/progenitor cells endowed with a high self-renewal ability and aberrant differentiation potential were able to give arise to the total tumor cell mass and generate the tumors with the phenotypic features resembling to original patient's melanomas [41,44-51,53,54].

Although this importance advance, future studies are essential for further establish the biomarkers of melanoma stem/progenitor cells and signaling pathways involved in the regulation of their malignant behavior *versus* their differentiated progenies. In this matter, we are reporting here the gene products that are frequently deregulated in melanoma cells during disease progression and which may constitute potential molecular biomarkers and therapeutic targets for improving the efficacy of diagnosis, prognosis and treatment of melanoma patients.

Novel Biomarkers for an Earlier Diagnosis and Effective Prognosis of Melanoma Patients

The clinical diagnosis of cutaneous melanomas at early stages retains a big challenge for the experimented pathologists and generally is made only after they become visible on skin. Moreover, a skin biopsy and different tumor imaging tests such as X-rays, computed tomography (CT) scan, magnetic resonance imaging (MRI) and positron emission tomography (PET) tests are often performed to definite the grades and stages of melanomas and screen for metastatic melanomas [55].

At the present time, few validated methods for an early detection of cutaneous melanomas and the establishment of the risk of the disease progression and relapse are available. Numerous microarray and histoimmunochemical analyses of different deregulated genes, detected in the malignant melanoma tissues and serum samples *versus* benign melanocytic naevi and normal tissues and serum samples have led to the identification of novel potential biomarkers for an earlier diagnosis and effective prognosis [15,20,35,56-64]. The potential biomarkers, alone or in combination, that may be used to establish the risk of disease progression and prognosis of melanoma patients include the detection in serum and/or malignant tissues of serum amyloid, MIC-1, VEGF, IL-8 and/or microphthalmia-associated transcription factor (MITF) [15,20,35,56-63]. More specifically, it has been observed that the MIC-1 cytokine was overexpressed in advanced and metastatic melanoma tissues and serum samples as compared to normal individuals [59,60]. Moreover, it has also been noted that the serum concentrations of diverse angiogenic factors such as VEGF, basic fibroblast factor (bFGF) and IL-8 were increased in melanoma patients relative to healthy individuals and associated with advanced stages and poor overall and progression-free survival of melanoma patients [15,20]. The results from another study carried out with thirty-five patients with stage IV melanoma have also indicated that 15 patients who responded to the chemotherapy showed a significant decrease in the serum IL-8 level while non-responders with progressive disease did not [64]. These data suggest that the detection of serum IL-8 level could serve as an indicator of the potential response of melanoma patients to the chemotherapy.

Hence, the assessment of the expression levels of these distinct biomarkers in melanoma tissue specimens and serum samples from patients in the clinics might represent novel screening tests for improving the current diagnostic and prognostic methods. Also, these novel biomarkers could be used to predict the potential response of melanoma patients to the inhibitory agents targeting these deregulated signaling elements, and thereby lead to an optimization of the choice for their therapeutic treatment.

Novel Therapeutic Strategies Against Aggressive, Metastatic and Recurrent Cutaneous Melanomas

The potential management of invasive, metastatic and/or relapsed melanomas may consist of metastasectomy, chemotherapy such as dacarbazine, alone or in combination with other chemotherapeutic drugs and radiotherapy without or plus stem cell-based transplantation therapies [1,2]. Moreover, certain patients with aggressive and incurable melanomas may also choose to enroll in novel clinical experimental trials with new treatments. In this matter, we are reporting recent therapeutic strategies that have been shown to be effective for eradicating the melanoma cells, counteracting tumor angiogenesis, suppressing growth and metastasis and which constitute promising approaches for improving the current therapies against aggressive, metastatic and recurrent melanomas.

Molecular Targeting of Melanoma Cells

Recent progress in melanoma research has led to the identification of several oncogenic signaling elements deregulated during melanoma initiation and progression to locally invasive and metastatic disease stages that constitute potential novel molecular therapeutic targets for eradicating the melanoma cells, including melanoma stem/progenitor cells, at primary and secondary neoplasms (Figure 1; Table 1). These deregulated gene products include B-Raf (V600E), N-Ras and c-KIT oncogenes, different RTKs such as EGFR, hepatocyte growth factor receptor c-MET and platelet-derived growth factor receptors (PDGF-Rs), sonic hedgehog, Wnt/β-catenin, Notch, Nodal/Cripto and hyaluronan (HA)/CD44 and their downstream signaling effectors such as PI3K/Akt, NF-kB and MIC-1 as well as ABC multidrug resistance transporters (Figure 1; Table 1) [10,14,19,60,65-86]. It has been shown that the targeting of these tumorigenic pathways and drug resistance-associated molecules may be effective for inhibiting the growth, invasion and/or metastases of melanoma cells *in vitro* and *in vivo* and improving the efficacy of current chemotherapeutric treatments [14,60,65-86]. For instance, it has been observed that an inhibitor of B-Raf (V600E), PLX4720 induced a cell cycle arrest and apoptosis exclusively in B-Raf (V600E)-melanoma cells and inhibited the tumor growth in B-Raf (V600E)-dependent tumor xenograft models without evidence of systemic toxicity [85].

In addition, the inhibition of EGFR tyrosine kinase activity by using a specific inhibitor, gefitinib has also been reported to suppress the proliferation of melanoma cells *in vitro* and tumor growth *in vivo* at least in part by inhibiting tumor angiogenesis [65-67]. Moreover, the molecular targeting of sonic hedgehog by using smoothened (SMO) co-receptor inhibitor, cyclopamine has been observed to prevent the growth, recurrence and metastasis of melanoma xenografts in mice *in vivo* [87]. Importantly, it has also been reported that the use of the monoclonal antibodies (mAbs) directed against stem cell-like marker CD133 induced cytotoxic effects in FEMX-I melanoma cells *in vitro* and decreased their metastatic capacity in a mouse model *in vivo* [50]. In the same way, the targeting ABCB5 efflux pump using mAb also inhibited the tumor growth of $CD133^{+}/ABCB5^{+}$ melanoma stem cell-derived xenografts *in vivo* [48].

Table 1. Potential molecular therapeutic targets in melanoma cells and their specific inhibitory agents

Targeted deregulated element	Name of inhibitory agent
mAb against stem cell-like surface marker:	
CD133	Anti-CD133 mAb
ABCB5	Anti-ABCB5 mAb
Growth factor signaling inhibitor:	
EGFR (erbB1) antibody	mAb-C225, cetuximab (IMC-C225), IMC-1121B
EGFR-TKI	Gefitinib, erlotinib, AG1478, PD153035
Anti-EGF antibody	ABX-EGF
Pan-erbB1/erbB2/erbB3/erbB4-TKI	Cl1033
Hedgehog	anti-SHH antibody, SMO inhibitor (cyclopamine, GDC-0449, BMS-833923, NVP-LDE225, IPI-926, IPI-269609)
Wnt/β-catenin	Anti-Wnt antibody, WIF-1
Notch	γ-secretase inhibitor (DAPT, MK-0752, GSI-18)
Nodal/Cripto	LEFTY, Anti-Cripto mAb
c-KIT	Imatinib mesylate, dasatinib
HA/CD44	Anti-CD44 mAb, soluble CD44 protein
VEGF	Anti-VEGF antibody (bevacizumab)
VEGFR-2	Anti-VEGFR-2 mAb (DC101)
VEGFR-2/EGFR/c-RET	Vandetanib (ZD6474)
ECM component/integrin	Anti-integrin antibody
Intracellular signaling inhibitor:	
B-Raf (V600E)	PLX 4032, PLX4720
PI3K	LY294002, rapamycin, CCL-779
NF-κB	IkBα inhibitor, sulfasalazine, bortezomib (PS-341) salinosporamides A (NPI-0052), parthenolide
COX-2	NS-396, etodolax, celecoxib, rofecoxib

DAPT, *N*-(N-3,5-difluorophenacetyl)-L-alanyl]-S-phenylglycine t-butyl ester; ECM, extracellular matrix; EGF, epidermal growth factor; EGFR, epidermal growth factor receptor; IkBα, inhibitor of nuclear factor-kBα; mAb, monoclonal antibody; NF-κB, nuclear factor-kappaB; PDGF-R, platelet-derived growth factor receptors; PI3K, phosphatidylinositol-3' kinase; SMO, smoothened; TKI, tyrosine kinase inhibitor; VEGF, vascular growth factor; VEGFR, vascular growth factor receptor; WIF-1, Wingless inhibitory factor-1 and Wnt, Wingless ligand.

Targeting of Local Tumor Microenvironment of Melanoma Cells

The use of cytotoxic agents targeting the tumor host cells such as myofibroblasts, bone marrow-derived cells, immune cells and/or endothelial cells constitutes the potential adjuvant therapeutic strategies of great promising to prevent or counteract the melanoma development, disease progression, metastases and disease relapse and improve the efficacy of current treatments. Several anti-angiogenic agents such as the specific inhibitors of VEGF/VEGFR system, thalidomine, angiostatin, endostatin and COX-2 inhibitors have been shown to inhibit the tumor growth, angiogenesis and metastases of melanoma cells at distant sites *in vitro* and *in vivo* (Table 1) [12,13,23,88,89]. For instance, it has been reported that the intratumorally or intravenously administration of a chimeric protein comprising abrin-a (ABRaA) toxin A-chain conjugated with human VEGF121 isoform substantially inhibited the tumor growth of B16-F10 murine melanoma cells subcutaneously implanted in C57Bl/6 mice [90]. Moreover, the vandetanib (ZD-6474), which is a potent and orally active pan-inhibitor of VEGFR-2, EGFR and c-RET tyrosine kinase activity, has also been shown to inhibit the tumor growth of melanoma cells and their extravasation and metastasis formation at distant sites in animal models *in vivo* [88,89]. The combined use of an anti-VEGFR-2 mAb DC101 plus anti-tyrosinase-related protein-1 (TYRP-1)/gp75 mAb TA99 has also been reported to induce a greater reduction of the tumor growth and lung metastasis derived from B16 mouse melanoma cells in mouse models *in vivo* as compared to the single agent treated and untreated animal groups [91]. Interestingly, it has also been reported that the down-regulation of the MIC-1 expression by small-interfering RNA reduced the melanoma tumorigenesis *in vivo* at least in part by inhibiting the angiogenic process [60].

Immunotherapies and Stem Cell-Based Therapies Against Aggressive and Metastatic Cutaneous Melanomas

Other promising approaches for the development of novel melanoma treatments include targeted immunotherapy, chemo-immunotherapies with immunosuppressive agents, immunotherapy-based melanoma vaccines such as the vaccination with *ex vivo*-generated and tumor antigen-loaded dendritic cells (DC), and stem cell-based and gene therapies (Table 1) [17,18,23,50,92-97]. In this matter, it has been reported that the melanoma stem cells can be efficiently targeted by using cancer testis antigens (CTA)-directed immunotherapeutic strategies [92].

In addition, since the systemic treatment of the melanoma patients with chemotherapeutic drugs might be accompanied by an increase of the inflammatory cytokine production by melanoma cells and recruitment of immune and BM-derived cells, the interference with the inflammatory and immune response also might represent a potential strategy to inhibit tumor angiogenesis and melanoma progression [23,98,99]. Consistently, it has been shown that the angiogenesis, tumorigenicity, and metastasis formation derived from subcutaneous and intravenous injections of highly metastatic A375SM human melanoma cells, respectively, were accelerated in *IFN-α/β receptor*$^{-/-}$ mice as compared wild-type mice suggesting an important role of endogenous IFN-α as suppressing agent of melanoma development [98]. Moreover, the blockade of adenosine receptor subtypes A2B and A3 has also been observed to result in a reduction of the expression levels and secretion of IL-8 and VEGF, respectively, in metastatic melanoma cells treated with etoposide (VP-16) and doxorubicin suggesting that the adenosine antagonists could be effective as chemosensibilizing agents [23]. It has also been reported that the mouse and human T cells engineered to express a chimeric antigen receptor (CAR) targeting VEGFR-2 mediated specific immune responses against VEGFR-2-expressing cells *in vitro*, and a combination of VEGFR-2 CAR-engineered mouse T cells plus IL-2 significantly inhibited the growth of vascularized tumors and prolonged the survival of mice *in vivo* [99].

Of particular therapeutic interest, diverse stem cell-based drug delivery systems have been developed to selectively target the metastatic melanoma cells that have spread at distant metastatic sites. For instance, it has been reported that the combined treatment with chemotherapeutic drug, 5-fluorocytosine (5FCyt) plus neural stem cells (NSCs) engineered for overexpressing the cytosine deaminase, which converts the non-cytotoxic pro-drug 5FCyt into its active metabolite 5-fluorouracil, resulted in a significant reduction in the tumor border in animal models with established melanoma brain metastasis *in vivo* [94].

Conclusions

Significant advancements made in few last years have provided important information on the gene products and molecular signaling pathways that are frequently deregulated in melanoma cells during melanoma formation and progression to locally advanced and metastatic disease stages. Consequently, these novel gene products constitute potential biomarkers and therapeutic targets for improving the accurate of current diagnostic and prognostic methods and efficacy of the therapeutic management of melanoma patients.

Acknowledgments

The authors on this work are supported in part by the U.S. Department of Defense (PC074289) and the National Institutes of Health National Cancer Institute (Grants CA78590, CA111294, CA131944, CA133774 and CA138791).

References

[1] Tsao H, Atkins MB, Sober AJ 2004 Management of cutaneous melanoma. *N Engl J Med* 351:998-1012

[2] Gray-Schopfer V, Wellbrock C, Marais R 2007 Melanoma biology and new targeted therapy. *Nature* 445:851-857

[3] Balch CM, Buzaid AC, Soong SJ, Atkins MB, Cascinelli N, Coit DG, Fleming ID, Gershenwald JE, Houghton A, Jr., Kirkwood JM, McMasters KM, Mihm MF, Morton DL, Reintgen DS, Ross MI, Sober A, Thompson JA, Thompson JF 2001 Final version of the American Joint Committee on Cancer staging system for cutaneous melanoma. *J Clin Oncol* 19:3635-3648

[4] Francken AB, Bastiaannet E, Hoekstra HJ 2005 Follow-up in patients with localised primary cutaneous melanoma. *Lancet Oncol* 6:608-621

[5] Bastiaannet E, Beukema JC, Hoekstra HJ 2005 Radiation therapy following lymph node dissection in melanoma patients: treatment, outcome and complications. *Cancer Treat Rev* 31:18-26

[6] Buzaid AC 2004 Management of metastatic cutaneous melanoma. *Oncology* (Williston Park) 18:1443-1450

[7] Danson S, Lorigan P 2005 Improving outcomes in advanced malignant melanoma: update on systemic therapy. *Drugs* 65:733-743

[8] Comis RL 1976 DTIC (NSC-45388) in malignant melanoma: a perspective. *Cancer Treat Rep* 60:165-176

[9] Hill GJ, Metter GE, Krementz ET, Fletcher WS, Golomb FM, Ramirez G, Grage TB, Moss SE 1979 DTIC and combination therapy for melanoma. II. Escalating schedules of DTIC with BCNU, CCNU, and vincristine. *Cancer Treat Rep* 63:1989-1992

[10] Tawbi HA, Buch SC 2010 Chemotherapy resistance abrogation in metastatic melanoma. *Clin Adv Hematol Oncol* 8:259-266

[11] Liu ZJ, Xiao M, Balint K, Smalley KS, Brafford P, Qiu R, Pinnix CC, Li X, Herlyn M 2006 Notch1 signaling promotes primary melanoma progression by activating mitogen-activated protein kinase/phosphatidylinositol 3-kinase-Akt pathways and up-regulating N-cadherin expression. *Cancer Res* 66:4182-4190

[12] Mehnert JM, McCarthy MM, Jilaveanu L, Flaherty KT, Aziz S, Camp RL, Rimm DL, Kluger HM 2010 Quantitative expression of VEGF, VEGF-R1, VEGF-R2, and VEGF-R3 in melanoma tissue microarrays. *Hum Pathol* 41:375-384

[13] Gangjee A, Kurup S, Ihnat MA, Thorpe JE, Shenoy SS 2010 Synthesis and biological activity of N(4)-phenylsubstituted-6-(2,4-dichloro phenylmethyl)-7H-pyrrolo[2,3-d]pyrimidine-2,4-diamines as vascular endothelial growth factor receptor-2 inhibitors and antiangiogenic and antitumor agents. *Bioorg Med Chem* 18:3575-3587

[14] Mimeault M, Bonenfant D, Batra SK 2004 New advances on the functions of epidermal growth factor receptor and ceramides in skin cell differentiation, disorders and cancers. *Skin Pharmacol Physiol* 17:153-166

[15] Rofstad EK, Halsor EF 2000 Vascular endothelial growth factor, interleukin 8, platelet-derived endothelial cell growth factor, and basic fibroblast growth factor promote angiogenesis and metastasis in human melanoma xenografts. *Cancer Res* 60:4932-4938

[16] Pinnix CC, Herlyn M 2007 The many faces of Notch signaling in skin-derived cells. *Pigment Cell Res* 20:458-465

[17] Mimeault M, Batra SK 2008 Targeting of cancer stem/progenitor cells plus stem cell-based therapies: the ultimate hope for treating and curing aggressive and recurrent cancers. *Panminerva Med* 50:3-18

[18] Mimeault M, Batra SK 2010 Recent advances on skin-resident stem/progenitor cell functions in skin regeneration, aging and cancers and novel anti-aging and cancer therapies. *J Cell Mol Med* 14:116-134

[19] Ohshima Y, Yajima I, Takeda K, Iida M, Kumasaka M, Matsumoto Y, Kato M 2010 c-RET molecule in malignant melanoma from oncogenic

RET-carrying transgenic mice and human cell lines. *PLoS ONE* 5:e10279

[20] Ugurel S, Rappl G, Tilgen W, Reinhold U 2001 Increased serum concentration of angiogenic factors in malignant melanoma patients correlates with tumor progression and survival. *J Clin Oncol* 19:577-583

[21] Frank NY, Schatton T, Kim S, Zhan Q, Wilson BJ, Ma J, Saab KR, Osherov V, Widlund HR, Gasser M, Waaga-Gasser AM, Kupper TS, Murphy GF, Frank MH 2011 VEGFR-1 expressed by malignant melanoma initiating cells is required for tumor growth. *Cancer Res*

[22] Ruiter D, Bogenrieder T, Elder D, Herlyn M 2002 Melanoma-stroma interactions: structural and functional aspects. *Lancet Oncol* 3:35-43

[23] Merighi S, Simioni C, Gessi S, Varani K, Mirandola P, Tabrizi MA, Baraldi PG, Borea PA 2009 A(2B) and A(3) adenosine receptors modulate vascular endothelial growth factor and interleukin-8 expression in human melanoma cells treated with etoposide and doxorubicin. *Neoplasia* 11:1064-1073

[24] Erb P, Ji J, Kump E, Mielgo A, Wernli M 2008 Apoptosis and pathogenesis of melanoma and nonmelanoma skin cancer. *Adv Exp Med Biol* 624:283-295

[25] Rass K, Reichrath J 2008 UV damage and DNA repair in malignant melanoma and nonmelanoma skin cancer. *Adv Exp Med Biol* 624:162-178

[26] Hussein MR 2005 Ultraviolet radiation and skin cancer: molecular mechanisms. *J Cutan Pathol* 32:191-205

[27] Pons M, Quintanilla M 2006 Molecular biology of malignant melanoma and other cutaneous tumors. *Clin Transl Onco*l 8:466-474

[28] Mimeault M, Batra SK 2009 Recent insights into the molecular mechanisms involved in aging and the malignant transformation of adult stem/progenitor cells and their therapeutic implications. *Ageing Res Rev* 8:94-112

[29] Ackermann J, Frutschi M, Kaloulis K, McKee T, Trumpp A, Beermann F 2005 Metastasizing melanoma formation caused by expression of activated N-RasQ61K on an INK4a-deficient background. *Cancer Res* 65:4005-4011

[30] Algazi AP, Soon CW, Daud AI 2010 Treatment of cutaneous melanoma: current approaches and future prospects. *Cancer Manag Res* 2:197-211

[31] Davies H, Bignell GR, Cox C, Stephens P, Edkins S, Clegg S, Teague J, Woffendin H, Garnett MJ, Bottomley W, Davis N, Dicks E, Ewing R, Floyd Y, Gray K, Hall S, Hawes R, Hughes J, Kosmidou V, Menzies A,

Mould C, Parker A, Stevens C, Watt S, Hooper S, Wilson R, Jayatilake H, Gusterson BA, Cooper C, Shipley J, Hargrave D, Pritchard-Jones K, Maitland N, Chenevix-Trench G, Riggins GJ, Bigner DD, Palmieri G, Cossu A, Flanagan A, Nicholson A, Ho JW, Leung SY, Yuen ST, Weber BL, Seigler HF, Darrow TL, Paterson H, Marais R, Marshall CJ, Wooster R, Stratton MR, Futreal PA 2002 Mutations of the BRAF gene in human cancer. *Nature* 417:949-954

[32] Curtin JA, Busam K, Pinkel D, Bastian BC 2006 Somatic activation of KIT in distinct subtypes of melanoma. *J Clin Oncol* 24:4340-4346

[33] Antonescu CR, Busam KJ, Francone TD, Wong GC, Guo T, Agaram NP, Besmer P, Jungbluth A, Gimbel M, Chen CT, Veach D, Clarkson BD, Paty PB, Weiser MR 2007 L576P KIT mutation in anal melanomas correlates with KIT protein expression and is sensitive to specific kinase inhibition. *Int J Cancer* 121:257-264

[34] Jonsson A, Tuominen R, Grafstrom E, Hansson J, Egyhazi S 2010 High frequency of p16(INK4A) promoter methylation in NRAS-mutated cutaneous melanoma. *J Invest Dermatol* 130:2809-2817

[35] Jonsson G, Busch C, Knappskog S, Geisler J, Miletic H, Ringner M, Lillehaug JR, Borg A, Lonning PE 2010 Gene expression profiling-based identification of molecular subtypes in stage IV melanomas with different clinical outcome. *Clin Cancer Res* 16:3356-3367

[36] Chin L 2003 The genetics of malignant melanoma: lessons from mouse and man. *Nat Rev Cancer* 3:559-570

[37] Tchernev G, Orfanos CE 2007 Downregulation of cell cycle modulators p21, p27, p53, Rb and proapoptotic Bcl-2-related proteins Bax and Bak in cutaneous melanoma is associated with worse patient prognosis: preliminary findings. *J Cutan Patho*l 34:247-256

[38] Kostov M, Mijovic Z, Mihailovic D, Cerovic S, Stojanovic M, Jelic M 2010 Correlation of cell cycle regulatory proteins (p53 and p16(ink)(a)) and bcl-2 oncoprotein with mitotic index and thickness of primary cutaneous malignant melanoma. *Bosn J Basic Med Sci* 10:276-281

[39] Monahan KB, Rozenberg GI, Krishnamurthy J, Johnson SM, Liu W, Bradford MK, Horner J, DePinho RA, Sharpless NE 2010 Somatic p16(INK4a) loss accelerates melanomagenesis. *Oncogene* 29:5809-5817

[40] Hansson J 2010 Familial cutaneous melanoma. *Adv Exp Med Biol* 685:134-145

[41] Fang D, Nguyen TK, Leishear K, Finko R, Kulp AN, Hotz S, Van Belle PA, Xu X, Elder DE, Herlyn M 2005 A tumorigenic subpopulation with stem cell properties in melanomas. *Cancer Res* 65:9328-9337

[42] Mimeault M, Batra SK 2006 Recent advances on the significance of stem cells in tissue regeneration and cancer therapies. *Stem Cells* 24:2319-2345

[43] Mimeault M, Hauke R, Mehta PP, Batra SK 2007 Recent advances on cancer stem/progenitor cell research: therapeutic implications for overcoming resistance to the most aggressive cancers. *J Mol Cell Med* 11:981-1011

[44] Frank NY, Margaryan A, Huang Y, Schatton T, Waaga-Gasser AM, Gasser M, Sayegh MH, Sadee W, Frank MH 2005 ABCB5-mediated doxorubicin transport and chemoresistance in human malignant melanoma. *Cancer Res* 65:4320-4333

[45] Dou J, Pan M, Wen P, Li Y, Tang Q, Chu L, Zhao F, Jiang C, Hu W, Hu K, Gu N 2007 Isolation and identification of cancer stem-like cells from murine melanoma cell lines. *Cell Mol Immunol* 4:467-472

[46] Monzani E, Facchetti F, Galmozzi E, Corsini E, Benetti A, Cavazzin C, Gritti A, Piccinini A, Porro D, Santinami M, Invernici G, Parati E, Alessandri G, La Porta CA 2007 Melanoma contains CD133 and ABCG2 positive cells with enhanced tumourigenic potential. *Eur J Cancer* 43:935-946

[47] Keshet GI, Goldstein I, Itzhaki O, Cesarkas K, Shenhav L, Yakirevitch A, Treves AJ, Schachter J, Amariglio N, Rechavi G 2008 MDR1 expression identifies human melanoma stem cells. *Biochem Biophys Res Commun* 368:930-936

[48] Schatton T, Murphy GF, Frank NY, Yamaura K, Waaga-Gasser AM, Gasser M, Zhan Q, Jordan S, Duncan LM, Weishaupt C, Fuhlbrigge RC, Kupper TS, Sayegh MH, Frank MH 2008 Identification of cells initiating human melanomas. *Nature* 451:345-349

[49] Grichnik JM, Burch JA, Schulteis RD, Shan S, Liu J, Darrow TL, Vervaert CE, Seigler HF 2006 Melanoma, a tumor based on a mutant stem cell? *J Invest Dermatol* 126:142-153

[50] Rappa G, Fodstad O, Lorico A 2008 The stem cell-associated antigen CD133 (Prominin-1) is a molecular therapeutic target for metastatic melanoma. *Stem Cells* 26:3008-3017

[51] Ma J, Lin JY, Alloo A, Wilson BJ, Schatton T, Zhan Q, Murphy GF, Waaga-Gasser AM, Gasser M, Stephen HF, Frank NY, Frank MH 2010 Isolation of tumorigenic circulating melanoma cells. *Biochem Biophys Res Commun* 402:711-717

[52] Fusi A, Reichelt U, Busse A, Ochsenreither S, Rietz A, Maisel M, Keilholz U 2011 Expression of the stem cell markers nestin and CD133 on circulating melanoma cells. *J Invest Dermatol* 131:487-494

[53] Boonyaratanakornkit JB, Yue L, Strachan LR, Scalapino KJ, LeBoit PE, Lu Y, Leong SP, Smith JE, Ghadially R 2010 Selection of tumorigenic melanoma cells using ALDH. *J Invest Dermatol* 130:2799-2808

[54] Boiko AD, Razorenova OV, van de Rijn M, Swetter SM, Johnson DL, Ly DP, Butler PD, Yang GP, Joshua B, Kaplan MJ, Longaker MT, Weissman IL 2010 Human melanoma-initiating cells express neural crest nerve growth factor receptor CD271. *Nature* 466:133-137

[55] Patnana M, Bronstein Y, Szklaruk J, Bedi DG, Hwu WJ, Gershenwald JE, Prieto VG, Ng CS 2011 Multimethod imaging, staging, and spectrum of manifestations of metastatic melanoma. *Clin Radiol* 66:224-236

[56] Ugurel S, Houben R, Schrama D, Voigt H, Zapatka M, Schadendorf D, Brocker EB, Becker JC 2007 Microphthalmia-associated transcription factor gene amplification in metastatic melanoma is a prognostic marker for patient survival, but not a predictive marker for chemosensitivity and chemotherapy response. *Clin Cancer Res* 13:6344-6350

[57] Matharoo-Ball B, Ratcliffe L, Lancashire L, Ugurel S, Miles AK, Weston DJ, Rees R, Schadendorf D, Ball G, Creaser CS 2007 Diagnostic biomarkers differentiating metastatic melanoma patients from healthy controls identified by an integrated MALDI-TOF mass spectrometry/bioinformatic approach. *Proteomics Clin Appl* 1:605-620

[58] Utikal J, Schadendorf D, Ugurel S 2007 Serologic and immunohistochemical prognostic biomarkers of cutaneous malignancies. *Arch Dermatol Res* 298:469-477

[59] Boyle GM, Pedley J, Martyn AC, Banducci KJ, Strutton GM, Brown DA, Breit SN, Parsons PG 2009 Macrophage inhibitory cytokine-1 is overexpressed in malignant melanoma and is associated with tumorigenicity. *J Invest Dermatol 1*29:383-391

[60] Huh SJ, Chung CY, Sharma A, Robertson GP 2010 Macrophage inhibitory cytokine-1 regulates melanoma vascular development. *Am J Pathol* 176:2948-2957

[61] Ugurel S, Thirumaran RK, Bloethner S, Gast A, Sucker A, Mueller-Berghaus J, Rittgen W, Hemminki K, Becker JC, Kumar R, Schadendorf D 2007 B-RAF and N-RAS mutations are preserved during short time in vitro propagation and differentially impact prognosis. *PLoS ONE* 2:e236

[62] Findeisen P, Zapatka M, Peccerella T, Matzk H, Neumaier M, Schadendorf D, Ugurel S 2009 Serum amyloid A as a prognostic marker

in melanoma identified by proteomic profiling. *J Clin Oncol* 27:2199-2208

[63] Busch C, Geisler J, Knappskog S, Lillehaug JR, Lonning PE 2010 Alterations in the p53 pathway and p16INK4a expression predict overall survival in metastatic melanoma patients treated with dacarbazine. *J Invest Dermatol* 130:2514-2516

[64] Brennecke S, Deichmann M, Naeher H, Kurzen H 2005 Decline in angiogenic factors, such as interleukin-8, indicates response to chemotherapy of metastatic melanoma. *Melanoma Res* 15:515-522

[65] Iivanainen E, Lauttia S, Zhang N, Tvorogov D, Kulmala J, Grenman R, Salven P, Elenius K 2009 The EGFR inhibitor gefitinib suppresses recruitment of pericytes and bone marrow-derived perivascular cells into tumor vessels. *Microvasc Res* 78:278-285

[66] Djerf EA, Trinks C, Abdiu A, Thunell LK, Hallbeck AL, Walz TM 2009 ErbB receptor tyrosine kinases contribute to proliferation of malignant melanoma cells: inhibition by gefitinib (ZD1839). *Melanoma Res* 19:156-166

[67] Amin DN, Bielenberg DR, Lifshits E, Heymach JV, Klagsbrun M 2008 Targeting EGFR activity in blood vessels is sufficient to inhibit tumor growth and is accompanied by an increase in VEGFR-2 dependence in tumor endothelial cells. *Microvasc Res* 76:15-22

[68] Chin L, Garraway LA, Fisher DE 2006 Malignant melanoma: genetics and therapeutics in the genomic era. *Genes Dev* 20:2149-2182

[69] Curtin JA, Busam K, Pinkel D, Bastian BC 2006 Somatic activation of KIT in distinct subtypes of melanoma. *J Clin Oncol* 24:4340-4346

[70] Guo Y, Ma J, Wang J, Che X, Narula J, Bigby M, Wu M, Sy MS 1994 Inhibition of human melanoma growth and metastasis in vivo by anti-CD44 monoclonal antibody. *Cancer Res* 54:1561-1565

[71] Ahrens T, Sleeman JP, Schempp CM, Howells N, Hofmann M, Ponta H, Herrlich P, Simon JC 2001 Soluble CD44 inhibits melanoma tumor growth by blocking cell surface CD44 binding to hyaluronic acid. *Oncogene* 20:3399-3408

[72] Weeraratna AT, Jiang Y, Hostetter G, Rosenblatt K, Duray P, Bittner M, Trent JM 2002 Wnt5a signaling directly affects cell motility and invasion of metastatic melanoma. *Cancer Cell* 1:279-288

[73] Smalley KS, Contractor R, Nguyen TK, Xiao M, Edwards R, Muthusamy V, King AJ, Flaherty KT, Bosenberg M, Herlyn M, Nathanson KL 2008 Identification of a novel subgroup of melanomas

with KIT/cyclin-dependent kinase-4 overexpression. *Cancer Res* 68:5743-5752

[74] Hodi FS, Friedlander P, Corless CL, Heinrich MC, Mac RS, Kruse A, Jagannathan J, Van den Abbeele AD, Velazquez EF, Demetri GD, Fisher DE 2008 Major response to imatinib mesylate in KIT-mutated melanoma. *J Clin Oncol* 26:2046-2051

[75] Bartolazzi A, Peach R, Aruffo A, Stamenkovic I 1994 Interaction between CD44 and hyaluronate is directly implicated in the regulation of tumor development. *J Exp Med* 180:53-66

[76] Knight LA, Di Nicolantonio F., Whitehouse P, Mercer S, Sharma S, Glaysher S, Johnson P, Cree IA 2004 The *in vitro* effect of gefitinib ('Iressa') alone and in combination with cytotoxic chemotherapy on human solid tumours. *BMC Cancer* 4:83

[77] Kim Y, Lee YS, Choe J, Lee H, Kim YM, Jeoung D 2008 CD44-epidermal growth factor receptor interaction mediates hyaluronic acid-promoted cell motility by activating protein kinase C signaling involving Akt, Rac1, Phox, reactive oxygen species, focal adhesion kinase, and MMP-2. *J Biol Chem* 283:22513-22528

[78] Qiu L, Wang Q, Di W, Jiang Q, Schefeller E, Derby S, Wanebo H, Yan B, Wan Y 2005 Transient activation of EGFR/AKT cell survival pathway and expression of survivin contribute to reduced sensitivity of human melanoma cells to betulinic acid. *Int J Oncol* 27:823-830

[79] Kumano K, Masuda S, Sata M, Saito T, Lee SY, Sakata-Yanagimoto M, Tomita T, Iwatsubo T, Natsugari H, Kurokawa M, Ogawa S, Chiba S 2008 Both Notch1 and Notch2 contribute to the regulation of melanocyte homeostasis. *Pigment Cell Melanoma Res* 21:70-78

[80] Postovit LM, Seftor EA, Seftor RE, Hendrix MJ 2007 Targeting Nodal in malignant melanoma cells. *Expert Opin Ther Targets* 11:497-505

[81] Postovit LM, Margaryan NV, Seftor EA, Hendrix MJ 2008 Role of nodal signaling and the microenvironment underlying melanoma plasticity. *Pigment Cell Melanoma Res* 21:348-357

[82] Nickoloff BJ, Hendrix MJ, Pollock PM, Trent JM, Miele L, Qin JZ 2005 Notch and NOXA-related pathways in melanoma cells. *J Investig Dermatol Symp Proc* 10:95-104

[83] Puri N, Ahmed S, Janamanchi V, Tretiakova M, Zumba O, Krausz T, Jagadeeswaran R, Salgia R 2007 c-Met is a potentially new therapeutic target for treatment of human melanoma. *Clin Cancer Res* 13:2246-2253

[84] Woodman SE, Trent JC, Stemke-Hale K, Lazar AJ, Pricl S, Pavan GM, Fermeglia M, Gopal YN, Yang D, Podoloff DA, Ivan D, Kim KB,

Papadopoulos N, Hwu P, Mills GB, Davies MA 2009 Activity of dasatinib against L576P KIT mutant melanoma: molecular, cellular, and clinical correlates. *Mol Cancer Ther* 8:2079-2085

[85] Tsai J, Lee JT, Wang W, Zhang J, Cho H, Mamo S, Bremer R, Gillette S, Kong J, Haass NK, Sproesser K, Li L, Smalley KS, Fong D, Zhu YL, Marimuthu A, Nguyen H, Lam B, Liu J, Cheung I, Rice J, Suzuki Y, Luu C, Settachatgul C, Shellooe R, Cantwell J, Kim SH, Schlessinger J, Zhang KY, West BL, Powell B, Habets G, Zhang C, Ibrahim PN, Hirth P, Artis DR, Herlyn M, Bollag G 2008 Discovery of a selective inhibitor of oncogenic B-Raf kinase with potent antimelanoma activity. *Proc Natl Acad Sci U S A* 105:3041-3046

[86] Halaban R, Zhang W, Bacchiocchi A, Cheng E, Parisi F, Ariyan S, Krauthammer M, McCusker JP, Kluger Y, Sznol M 2010 PLX4032, a selective BRAF(V600E) kinase inhibitor, activates the ERK pathway and enhances cell migration and proliferation of BRAF melanoma cells. *Pigment Cell Melanoma Res* 23:190-200

[87] Stecca B, Mas C, Clement V, Zbinden M, Correa R, Piguet V, Beermann F, Ruiz IA 2007 Melanomas require HEDGEHOG-GLI signaling regulated by interactions between GLI1 and the RAS-MEK/AKT pathways. P*roc Natl Acad Sci U S A* 104:5895-5900

[88] Wedge SR, Ogilvie DJ, Dukes M, Kendrew J, Chester R, Jackson JA, Boffey SJ, Valentine PJ, Curwen JO, Musgrove HL, Graham GA, Hughes GD, Thomas AP, Stokes ES, Curry B, Richmond GH, Wadsworth PF, Bigley AL, Hennequin LF 2002 ZD6474 inhibits vascular endothelial growth factor signaling, angiogenesis, and tumor growth following oral administration. *Cancer Res* 62:4645-4655

[89] Kusters B, Kats G, Roodink I, Verrijp K, Wesseling P, Ruiter DJ, de Waal RM, Leenders WP 2007 Micronodular transformation as a novel mechanism of VEGF-A-induced metastasis. *Oncogene* 26:5808-5815

[90] Smagur A, Boyko MM, Biront NV, Cichon T, Szala S 2009 Chimeric protein ABRaA-VEGF121 is cytotoxic towards VEGFR-2-expressing PAE cells and inhibits B16-F10 melanoma growth. *Acta Biochim Pol* 56:115-124

[91] Patel D, Bassi R, Hooper AT, Sun H, Huber J, Hicklin DJ, Kang X 2008 Enhanced suppression of melanoma tumor growth and metastasis by combined therapy with anti-VEGF receptor and anti-TYRP-1/gp75 monoclonal antibodies. *Anticancer Res* 28:2679-2686

[92] Sigalotti L, Covre A, Zabierowski S, Himes B, Colizzi F, Natali PG, Herlyn M, Maio M 2008 Cancer testis antigens in human melanoma

stem cells: Expression, distribution, and methylation status. *J Cell Physiol* 215:287-291

[93] den Brok MH, Nierkens S, Figdor CG, Ruers TJ, Adema GJ 2005 Dendritic cells: tools and targets for antitumor vaccination. *Expert Rev Vaccines* 4:699-710

[94] Aboody KS, Bush RA, Garcia E, Metz MZ, Najbauer J, Justus KA, Phelps DA, Remack JS, Yoon KJ, Gillespie S, Kim SU, Glackin CA, Potter PM, Danks MK 2006 Development of a tumor-selective approach to treat metastatic cancer. *PLoS ONE* 1:e23

[95] Dubsky P, Saito H, Leogier M, Dantin C, Connolly JE, Banchereau J, Palucka AK 2007 IL-15-induced human DC efficiently prime melanoma-specific naive CD8+ T cells to differentiate into CTL. *Eur J Immunol* 37:1678-1690

[96] Sotomayor MG, Yu H, Antonia S, Sotomayor EM, Pardoll DM 2002 Advances in gene therapy for malignant melanoma. *Cancer Control* 9:39-48

[97] Mimeault M, Batra SK 2010 New promising drug targets in cancer- and metastasis-initiating cells. *Drug Discov Today* 15:354-364

[98] McCarty MF, Bielenberg D, Donawho C, Bucana CD, Fidler IJ 2002 Evidence for the causal role of endogenous interferon-alpha/beta in the regulation of angiogenesis, tumorigenicity, and metastasis of cutaneous neoplasms. *Clin Exp Metastasis* 19:609-615

[99] Chinnasamy D, Yu Z, Theoret MR, Zhao Y, Shrimali RK, Morgan RA, Feldman SA, Restifo NP, Rosenberg SA 2010 Gene therapy using genetically modified lymphocytes targeting VEGFR-2 inhibits the growth of vascularized syngenic tumors in mice. *J Clin Invest* 120:3953-3968

In: Metastatic Melanoma
Editors: S.A. Klein and J.P. Beckler
ISBN 978-1-61209-915-6

Chapter VII

"Melanoma Inhibitory Activity" (MIA) as a Serological Marker in Metastatic Uveal Melanoma

I. W. Reiniger**, *A. Kampik and U. C. Schaller
Department of Ophthalmology, Ludwig-Maximilians-University, Mathildenstr. 8, 80336 Munich, Germany

Abstract

Purpose: Uveal melanomas typically metastasize to the liver. A sensitive and specific serological marker for metastatic disease would be of great value. The small globular protein "melanoma inhibitory activity" (MIA) is established as a marker for cutaneous melanoma. This study was performed to evaluate MIA as potential serological marker for early detection of metastatic disease in uveal melanoma.

Method: In a prospective study, we collected serum samples of 390 patients with uveal melanoma. Serum samples were analysed by using a one-step enzyme-linked immunosorbent assay (ELISA) to quantify the MIA serum levels. All patients also underwent standardized A-scan echography to measure the maximum tumor height.

* Corresponding author: I. W. Reiniger, Department of Ophthalmology, Ludwig-Maximilians-University, Mathildenstr. 8, 80336 Munich. E-mail: ingrid.reiniger@med.uni-muenchen.de; Tel: (+49) 89 5160 3811; Fax: (+49) 89 5160 5160.

Results: 31 (7.9 %) patients had proven metastatic disease. The mean serum concentration of MIA in these patients was 17.22 ng/ml, whereas in the 359 patients without metastasis, 6.74 ng/ml ($p < 0.001$). Sixteen of the 31 patients presented with metastatic disease during follow-up. These patients showed a MIA of 6.49 ng/ml before and of 17.44 ng/ml after the development of metastasis ($p = 0.001$). Comparing different apical tumor thickness to MIA serum concentrations in patients without metastasis, no significant correlation was found. A correlation between local therapy and MIA serum concentrations could neither be seen.

Conclusion: The statistically highly significant elevation of MIA serum levels in patients with metastatic disease from melanoma suggests a promising role as a serum marker for monitoring these patients.

Introduction

Uveal melanoma is the most common primary intraocular malignancy in adults, affecting 6 to 8 persons per million each year in the western world [8, Figure 1]. This tumor is among the few types of cancer that are regularly treated before tissue can be examined and graded histologically to indicate the likehood of metastasis [16-18]. It is well recognized that the metastatic potential of uveal melanoma is not uniform. The 5-year mortality rates are 16% for patients with small tumors, 32% for medium tumors and 53% for those with large choroidal melanomas [6]. If metastatic disease develops the survival significantly decreases to less than a year [1].

Uveal melanomas typically metastasize to the liver. Patients are screened for metastasis on a semiannual basis using numerous liver function tests (LFTs) and imaging techniques [14,20]. Retrospective evaluations of screening tests showed a sensitivity per test ranging from 1.9 % for bilirubin to 25 % for alkaline phosphatase; specificity ranged from 86 % to 99 %, respectively. Both sensitivity and specificity of LFTs improved with the use of multiple tests [9,12]. Imaging tests were found to be highly specific but lacked sensitivity. The Collaborative Ocular Melanoma Study Group (COMS) followed prospectively a large series of patients with choroidal melanoma and evaluated systematically using a standard protocol to screen for metastatic spread: semi-annual LFTs should be included, liver ultrasonography and chest x-ray are recommended at the baseline only, given their findings of low sensitivity for both tests [7].

A more sensitive and, moreover, specific serological marker for metastatic disease would be of great value.

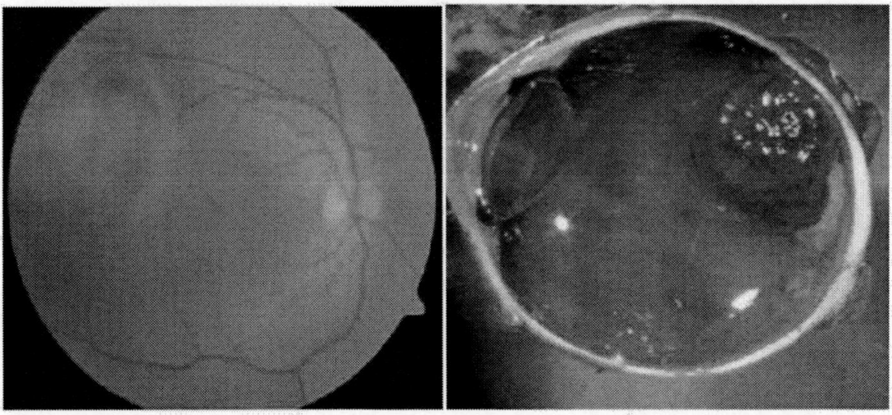

Figure 1. A) Clinical photography of a uveal melanoma (from: Photo Archive, Department of Ophthalmology, LMU, Munich). The lesion touches the temporal upper arc. B) Macroscopic histopathology after enucleation (from: Histology Archive, Department of Ophthalmology, LMU, Munich).

The protein S 100β is an important clinical marker for skin melanoma. In contrast, uveal melanomas express S 100β protein less frequently and to a lesser degree. As a serological marker, S 100β does not seem to be beneficial [13]. In contrast, the marker 5-S-cysteinyldopa has been shown to be useful, but its assessment is difficult and expensive [11].

Recently, the small globular protein melanoma inhibitory activity (MIA) was identified from tissue culture supernatant of melanoma cells in vitro by its ability to inhibit thymidine incorporation by melanoma cell lines [2]. MIA was then found to be specifically expressed by malignant melanoma cells, chondrocytes and a subgroup of advanced breast cancer [3-4]. This indicates a highly restricted expression pattern. Subsequently MIA was found to be a highly sensitive and specific serum marker for systemic cutaneous melanomas. In clinical studies, MIA serum levels correlate with the clinical tumor stage in melanoma patients, providing an enzyme-linked immunosorbent assay (Roche Diagnostics, Manheim, Germany) to monitor therapy and progression of this disease [3,5].

This study was performed to evaluate MIA serum levels in a large group of patients with uveal melanoma and its relevance as a serological serum marker for the screening for metastatic disease.

Materials and Methods

From November 1997 to December 2005 we consecutively collected and evaluated serum samples from 390 patients with uveal melanoma. Patients were recruited in the outpatient clinic of the Department of Ophthalmology of the Ludwig-Maximilians-University, Munich, Germany. All patients gave their informed consent prior to their inclusion in the study.

All patients underwent a complete ophthalmological examination including visual acuity testing, slitlamp examination, intraocular pressure and funduscopy. Fundus photographs were taken from all patients at each visit. Furthermore, we performed standardized A-scan echography to measure the maximum tumor height as described by Ossoinig [19]. The patients were screened for metastatic disease by using liver ultrasound and liver enzymes (alkaline phosphatase, AST, ALT).

Samples were obtained at each examination by drawing 5 ml venous blood into a sterile container containing lithium-heparin (Monovette, Sarsted AG und Co., 51588 Nünbrecht, Germany). Samples were then centrifuged for 15 minutes with 90000 turns per minute (Hettich, Universal, Tuttlingen, Germany). One ml serum was then removed and injected into another sterile container. Serum samples were evaluated in the Laboratory for Allergy, Dermatological Department of the Technical University in Munich, Germany. A one-step enzyme-linked immunosorbent assay (ELISA) was used to quantify the MIA serum levels (MIA-ELISA, Roche, Mannheim, Germany). The ELISA was performed as described by the manufacturer. Briefly, two monoclonal antibodies directed against the NH_2-terminal (clone 2F7) conjugated to horseradish peroxidase and against the COOH-terminal region (clone 1A12) conjucated to biotin, respectively, were used. Ten μl of serum or standard (Roche, included in the MIA-ELISA, recombinant MIA purified from transfected Chinese hamster ovary cells) were incubated with 200 μl reagent containing both antibodies in streptavidin-coated 96-well plates for 45 min with shaking. After washing three times with washing buffer (Roche, supplied with the MIA-ELISA), 200 μl of 2.2-azino-de- (3-ethylbenz-thiazoline sulphonate, Roche) was incubated in the wells for 30 min and measured colormetrically at 405 nm. Using the indicated standard concentrations linear signals were measured at MIA concentrations between 0.1 and 50 ng / ml. The reproducibility of this ELISA has been demonstrated previously [3].

Statistical analysis was performed using the Kruskall-Wallis-Test. Data were collected and analysed using Microsoft Excel and SPSS 11.0 for Windows.

Results

Two hundred and eight (53.4 %) of the patients were female and 182 (46.6 %) male. Patient's age varied from 23 to 96 years (median 62 years). The median duration of follow-up was 552 days (range: 17 days – 7.6 years).

From our 390 patients, 31 (7.9 %) had proven metastatic disease. The mean serum concentration of MIA in these patients was 17.22 ng/ml, whereas in the 359 patients without metastasis, 6.74 ng/ml. The difference in MIA serum levels between patients with and without overt metastatic disease was statistically highly significant ($p < 0.001$). Figure 2 shows a comparison between these two groups of patients. Note that the serum levels of patients with metastasis are far more scattered than the serum levels of patients without metastatic disease.

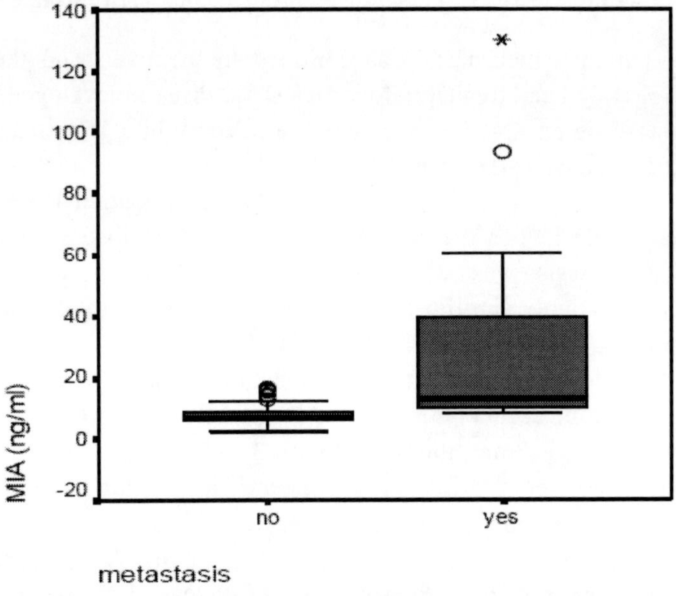

Figure 2. MIA serum levels in patients with vs. without metastasis. This difference was statistically highly significant ($p < 0.001$). Note that MIA levels of patients with proven metastasis were far more scattered.

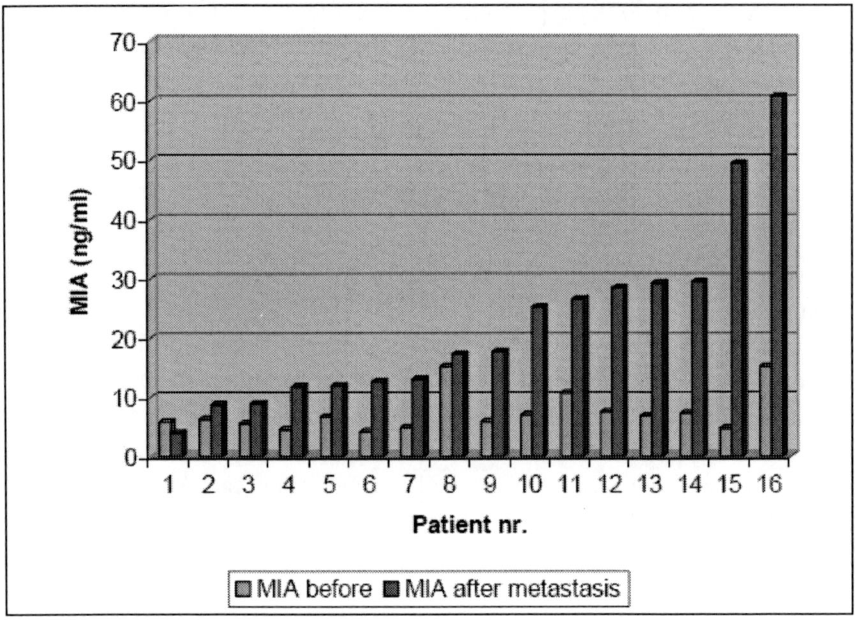

Figure 3. MIA level variation in the sixteen patients who developed metastasis during observation. This difference was also statistically highly significant ($p = 0.001$).

In our patients, metastasis was confined to the liver, and the primary tumor had already been treated before metastatic disease developed. No other sites of metastasis except the liver were detected. While 15 patients already presented with metastatic disease at initial presentation, metastasis were detected in 16 patients during observation. Of these 16 patients, we evaluated MIA serum levels before the appearance of metastatic disease (6.49 ng/ml) and after metastasis was detected (17.44 ng/ml). This difference was statistically also highly significant ($p = 0.001$). Figure 3 shows this subgroup of patients and the fluctuation in MIA serum levels.

We subdivided the group of patients without metastasis (359) according to different apical tumor thickness and compared MIA serum concentrations in the group of tumors < 3mm, tumors between 3 and 5 mm and tumors > 5 mm. Table 1 shows the median MIA serum concentrations in the three groups. The difference between these groups was statistically not significant ($p > 0.9$).

Also in the group of patients without metastatic disease, 189 patients had received a treatment of the primary tumor, 170 were followed periodically without treatment of the lesion, as no tumor growth was noted echographically. Table 1 compares MIA serum concentrations between patients who received a local therapy and those who were not treated for primary tumor. There was no significant difference in the serum levels between these two groups ($p > 0.6$).

Table 1. MIA concentrations according to different apical tumor thickness and local tumor therapy (in the group of patients without metastasis)

	all patients	max. apical tumor thickness			local therapy	
MIA (ng/ml)		< 3 mm	3-5 mm	> 5 mm	No (n=170)	Yes (n=189)
median	6.7	6.6	6.93	6.76	6.75	6.74
min	2.09	2.51	2.09	2.68	3.22	2.09
max	17.74	17.47	17.74	16.12	16.87	15.49

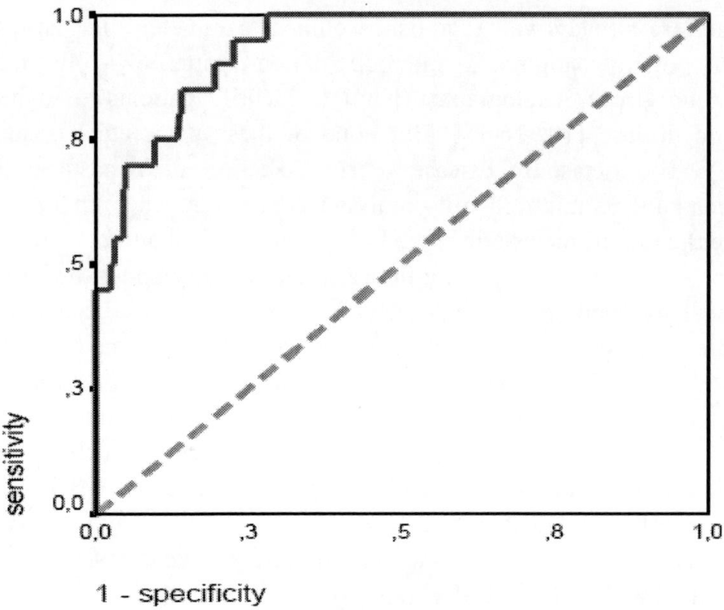

Figure 4. The preliminary ROC curve indicates that the protein MIA is a sensitive and specific test for the detection of metastatic disease in patients with uveal melanoma. The level of sensitivity was 90 % and of specificity 80.6 %, given a normal MIA level of 8.98 ng/ml.

To give an overview about sensitivity and specificity of MIA, we analysed the serum levels of patients with and without metastasis in a Receiver-Operating-Characteristics-curve (ROC). Figure 4 shows our ROC curve (continued line): The diagonal line (discontinued line) represents a 50 % level of sensitivity and specificity.

A diagnosis test can be considered significant, if the ROC curve diverges from the diagonal line. Another measure for quality of a diagnosis test is the area under the ROC curve (AUC). In our study, the AUC was 0.937 (CI 95 %: 0.897-0.977), and this was highly statistically significant ($p < 0.001$). Our ROC curve has a preliminary character, as 31 patients with metastasis are still not enough to give significant qualitative information. It would be necessary to have a minimum of 50 patients in each group, so that one patient doesn't correspond to more than 2 % of all patients [15].

Conclusion

There are already well established clinical parameters like largest tumor diameter, orange pigment, microcirculation pattern in the Confocal Indocyanine Green Angiography (ICG) to identify patients at high risk for metastatic disease [10, 16-18]. But none of these parameters is suitable to indicate early metastatic disease. Early detection of metastasis in uveal melanoma patients might identify individuals at a time when intervention may decrease the rate of metastatic spread or extend survival and may also help the patient and the family in planning future medical and personal care [7,24].

A sensitive and specific serological marker for metastatic disease would be of great value. In recent years, a new and more promising attachment-regulating protein, MIA, has been shown to be a tumor marker for cutaneous melanomas [2-5]. MIA interacts with components of the extracellular matrix, such as laminin and fibronectin, and is involved in cellular motility, metastasis, and modulation of immune responses. Therefore, MIA may have a function in regulating detachment of melanoma and possibly other cells from the extracellular matrix, which is an important step in metastasis [3].

An immunohistochemically positive MIA expression in primary and metastatic lesions of uveal melanoma could already be demonstrated [23]. Our study group could also demonstrate elevated MIA serum levels in patients with overt metastatic disease [21-23]. In the current study we evaluated MIA as a possible serum marker for uveal melanoma in a larger group of patients.

Our observations demonstrated that increased MIA serum levels depend on the metastatic progress of uveal melanoma as patients with metastatic uveal melanoma showed significantly elevated MIA serum levels. Interestingly, the serum levels of patients with metastatic disease were far more scattered than the serum levels of patients without metastasis. At present, we do not have a sufficient explanation for this observation, but one might hypothesize, that the scatter of serum levels represents variations in MIA expression. All our 31 patients with metastatic disease had a diffuse liver disease, making a correlation between MIA serum levels and size or number of metastases impossible.

Our data showed no statistical difference in the MIA serum levels between small, medium and large tumors in patients without metastatic disease. Also, we found no significant difference between treated and untreated patients. We conclude that local factors such as maximal apical tumor thickness and local therapy of the primary tumor do not influence MIA serum levels. As described for other tumor markers in medicine, MIA is not adequate to diagnose or stage a primary tumor.

It is also important to understand that the protein MIA is not a predictive marker, and therefore not useful to estimate the risk of developing metastatic disease. In other words, in melanoma patients showing normal MIA levels, future metastasis cannot be excluded. In contrast, an abnormal MIA serum level indicates the likely presence of metastatic disease and warrants careful screening.

In order to evaluate the sensitivity and specificity of a diagnostic test a Receiver-Operating-Characteristics-curve (ROC) is of great value. In this analysis, the quality of a diagnostic test is estimated by the area under the curve (AUC). In our study, the AUC was statistically highly significant. As mentioned before our ROC curve has a preliminary character, and the recruitment of further patients is required to give significant qualitative information.

As patients after development of metastatic disease were treated by dermatologists or oncologists not returning to the eye clinic, we lost contact to many patients. This is one reason why we do not have enough data about MIA as a parameter for therapy monitoring during chemotherapy. However, our data suggest that MIA is a useful screening parameter for detecting patients with metastatic uveal melanoma and that this protein may be valuable in the future. We hope to introduce MIA as a serological tumor marker for metastatic uveal melanoma in the clinical routine. Additionally, MIA could play an important role in the future in testing, introducing and monitoring new treatment options for metastatic uveal melanoma.

References

[1] Albert DM, Niffeneger AS, Willson JK (1992). Treatment of metastatic uveal melanoma: Review and recommendations. *Surv. Ophthalmol.* 36: 429-38.

[2] Blesch A, Bosserhoff AK, Apfel R, Behl C, Heßdörfer B, Schmitt A, Jachimczak P, Lottspeich F, Buettner R, Bogdahn U (1994). Cloning of a novel Malignant Melanoma-derived Growth-Regulatory Protein, MIA. *Cancer Res.* 54: 5695-701.

[3] Bosserhoff AK, Golob M, Buettner R, Landthaler M, Hein R (1998). MIA („melanoma inhibitory activity"): Biologische Funktionen und klinische Relevanz beim malignen Melanom. *Hautarzt.* 49: 762-9.

[4] Bosserhoff AK, Moser M, Hein R, Landthaler M, Buettner R (1999). In Situ Expression Patterns of Melanoma-Inhibiting activity (MIA) in: Melanomas and Breast Cancers. *J. Pathol.* 187: 446-54.

[5] Bosserhoff AK, Hauschild A, Hein R, Schadendorf D, Stockflesh E, Bogenrieder T, Landthaler M, Buettner R, Stolz W (2000). Elevated MIA serum levels are of relevance for management of metastasized malignant melanomas: results of a German multicenter study. *J. Invest. Dermatol.* 114(2):395-6.

[6] Diener-West M, Hawkins BS, Markowitz JA, Schachat AP (1992). A review of mortality from choroidal melanoma. A meta-analysis of 5-year mortality rates following enucleation. 1966 through 1988. *Arch. Ophthalmol.* 110: 245-50.

[7] Diener-West M, Reynolds SM, Agugliaro DJ, Caldwell R, Cumming K, Earle JD, Green DL, Hawkins BS, Hayman J, Jaiyesimi I, Kirkwood JM, Koh WJ, Robertson DM, Shaw JM, Thoma J; Collaborative ocular melanoma study group Report 23 (2004). Screening for metastasis from choroidal melanoma: the collaborative ocular melanoma study group Report 23. *J. Clin. Oncology.* 22: 2438-44.

[8] Egan KM, Seddon JM, Glynn RJ, Gragoudas ES, Albert DM (1988). Epidemiological aspects of uveal melanoma. *Surv. Ophthalmol.* 32: 239-51.

[9] Eskelin S, Pyrhonen S, Summanen P, Prause JU, Kivela T (1999). Screening for Metastatic Malignant Melanoma of the Uvea Revisited. *Cancer.* 85: 1151-9.

[10] Folberg R, Mehaffey M, Gardner LM, Meyer M, Rummelt V, Pe'er J (1997). The microcirculation of choroidal and ciliary body melanomas. *Eye.* 11: 227-38.

[11] Goto H, Tenou T, Kudo H, Iwasaki T, Maramatsu R, Usui M, Wakamatsu K, Ito S (1998). 5-S-Cysteinyldopa as a diagnostic tumor marker for uveal melanoma. *Nippon Ganka Gakkai Zasshi.* 102: 319-26.

[12] Hicks C, Foss AJE, Hungerford JL (1998). Predictive power of screening tests for metastasis in uveal melanoma. *Eye.* 12: 945-8.

[13] Kan-Mitchell J, Liggett PE, Taylor CR, Rao N, Granada ESV, Danenberg KD, White WL, Van Eldik LJ, Horikoshi T, Danenberg PV (1993). Differential S100ß Expression in Choroidal and Skin Melanomas: Quantitation by the Polymerase Chain Reaction. *Invest. Ophthalmol. Vis. Sci.* 34: 3366-75.

[14] Kuan AK, Jackson FI, Hanson J (1988). Multimodality detection of metastatic melanoma. *J. R. Soc. Med.* 81: 579-82.

[15] Metz CE (1978). Basic principles of ROC analysis. *Seminars in Nuclear Medicine.* 8: 283-98.

[16] Mooy CM, De Jong PTVM (1996). Prognostic Parameters in Uveal Melanoma: A Review. *Surv. Ophthalmol.* 41: 215-28.

[17] Mueller AJ, Bartsch DU, Schaller UC, Freeman WR, Kampik A (2001). Imaging the microcirculation of untreated and treated human choroidal melanomas. *Ophthalmology.* 23: 385-93.

[18] Mueller AJ, Freeman WR, Schaller UC, Kampik A, Folberg R (2002). Complex Microcirculation Patterns Detected by Confocal Indocyanine Green Angiography Predict Time to Growth of Small Choroidal Melanocytic Tumors. *Ophthalmology.* 109: 2207-14.

[19] Ossoinig KC, Bigar F, Kaefring SL (1975). Malignant melanoma of the choroid and the ciliary body: differential diagnosis in clinical echography. *Ultrasonography in ophthalmology*, Basel, Karger 83: 141-54.

[20] Pach JM, Robertson DM (1986). Metastasis from untreated uveal melanomas. *Arch. Ophthalmol.* 104: 1624-5.

[21] Reiniger IW, Schaller UC, Haritoglou C, Hein R, Bosserhoff AK, Kampik A, Mueller AJ (2005). "Melanoma inhibitory activity" (MIA): a promising serological tumour marker in metastatic uveal melanoma. *Graefes Arch. Clin. Exp. Ophthalmol.* 243 (11):1161-6.

[22] Schaller UC, Mueller AJ, Bosserhoff AK, Haraida S, Löhrs U, Buettner R, Kampik A (2000). Melanoma inhibitory activity (MIA): Evaluierung eines neuen tumorassoziierten Antigens als Serummarker für uveale Melanome. *Ophthalmologe* 97: 429-32.

[23] Schaller UC, Bosserhoff AK, Neubauer AS, Buettner R, Kampik A, Mueller AJ (2002). Melanoma inhibitory activity: a novel serum marker for uveal melanoma. *Melanoma Research.* 12: 593-9.

[24] Terheyden P, Kämpgen E, Rünger TM, Bröcker EB, Becker JC (1998). Immunochemotherapie des metastasierenden Uveamelanoms mit Interferon-α2b, Interleukin-2 und Fotemustin: Kasuistiken und Literaturübersicht. *Hautarzt.* 49: 770-3.

Index

A

B

C

D

E

F

K

L

M

N

Q

R

S

T

U

V

W

X

Z